50 ANTI-INFLAMMATORY RECIPES THAT ARE WORTH TRYING

Provides a Delicious and Satisfying 50 Day Anti-Inflammation Meal Plan That Has Been Optimized to Help Reduce Inflammation and to Keep You Feeling Healthy and Well-Balanced.

Gourmet LifeStyle

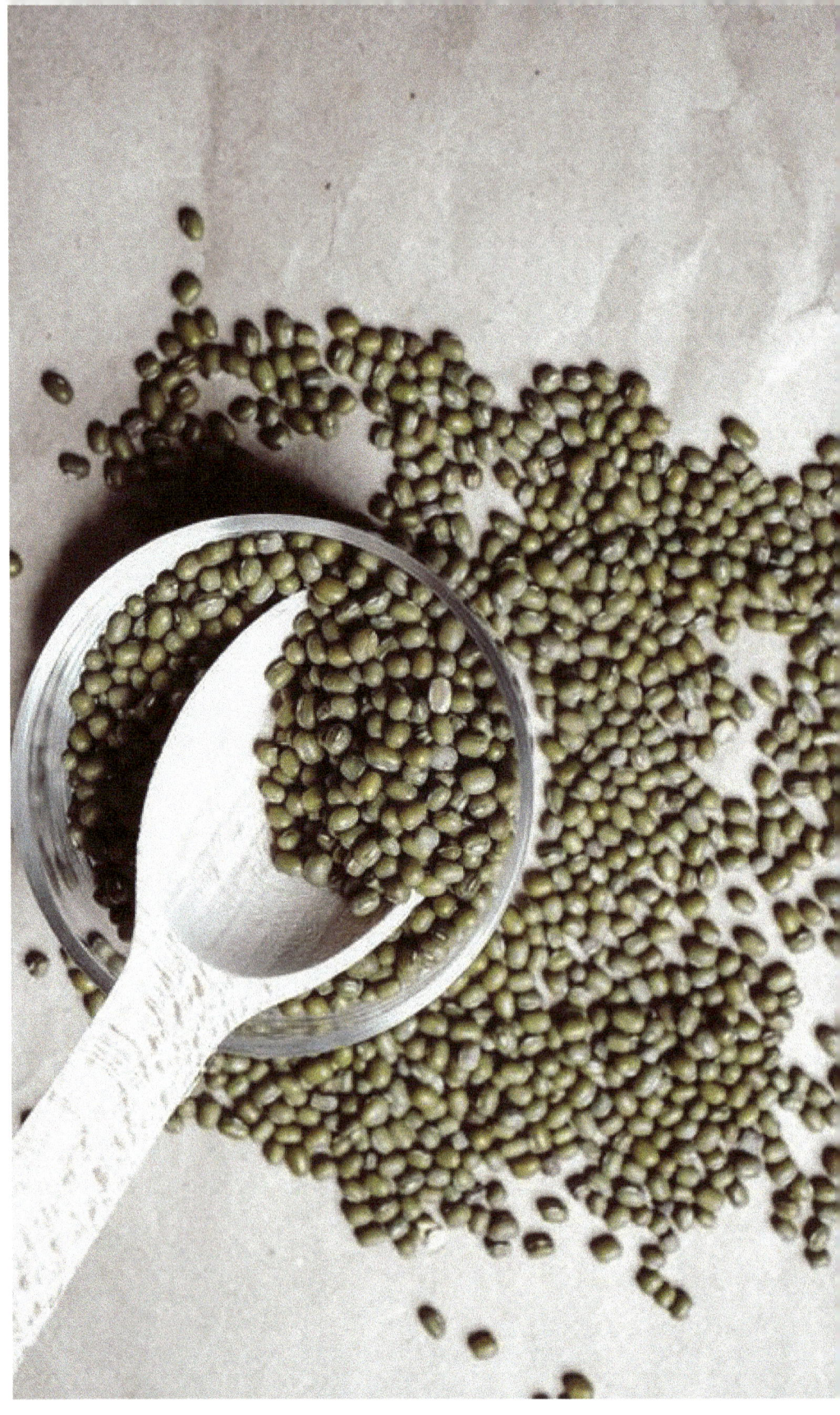

Table of Contents

INTRODUCTION

What is the Anti-Inflammatory Diet?

The anti-inflammatory diet is the best choice for your health if you have conditions that cause inflammation. Such conditions are asthma, chronic peptic ulcer, tuberculosis, rheumatoid arthritis, periodontitis, Crohn's disease, sinusitis, active hepatitis, etc. Along with medical treatment, proper nutrition is very important. An anti-inflammatory diet can help to reduce the pain from inflammation. Such a diet isn't a panacea but a significant help in any treatment.

Inflammation is a natural response of your body to infections, injuries, and illnesses. The classic symptoms of inflammation are redness, pain, heat, and swelling. Nevertheless, some diseases such as diabetes, heart disease, and cancer don't display any symptoms. That's why it's important to take preventive measures to protect your health.

The anti-inflammatory diet helps to enrich the organism with antioxidants which help reduce the level of free radicals in our bodies. The most common question that people ask is what to eat on the anti-inflammatory diet. It is actually a varied diet that includes many fruits, vegetables, whole grains, plant-based proteins (legumes and nuts), fatty fish, spices, condiments, and dressings. The only condition that should be followed is that all food should be organic. The most popular vegetables and fruits on the anti-inflammatory diet are leafy greens, cherries, raspberries, blackberries, tomatoes, cucumbers, etc. It also includes oatmeal, brown rice, and all grains that are high in fiber. Herbs and spices are natural antioxidants that will boost your health and flavor your food. You should avoid highly processed food (sugary drinks, chocolate, ice cream, French fries, burgers, sausages, deli meats), and overly greasy food. One more factor that will help is to make sure that you drink the correct amount of water per day. This helps to cleanse the body. There are a lot of apps that will help you track your water intake.

The anti-inflammatory diet is simple to follow, flexible, and not very strict. Nevertheless, there are some cons to be aware of. The anti-inflammatory diet can be costly as it calls for organic food. Likewise, it contains a lot of allergens such as nuts, seeds, and soy, which can cause problems for some people.

However, eating the right food will help to eliminate the cons of the diet. It is highly recommended to consult your doctor and get a complete medical examination before starting the diet. By doing this, you can avoid exacerbations and unwanted effects.

This is the most important information that you should know before starting a diet. No diet is a magic remedy for all diseases; it is simply a support for the body during treatment. Start your new healthy life from one small step and you will see the huge results within half a year. You can be sure that your body will be thankful to you by giving you a fresh look and energy for new achievements.

What to Eat and Avoid on the Anti-Inflammatory Diet

Meat, Poultry and Fish

The best choice for an anti-inflammatory diet is fish and seafood. This type of food is rich in omega-3 fatty acids with almost no allergic reactions. Meat can be eaten in moderation, although it is recommended to eat grass-fed meat.

What to eat	Eat occasionally	What to avoid
Tuna	Beef	Lamb
Sole	Chicken	Lard
Shrimps	Pork loin	Bacon
Turkey	Pork tenderloin	All remaining pork pieces
Halibut		
Trout		Breaded fish
Salmon		
Flounder		

Mackerel		
Oysters		
Sardines		
Catfish		
Clams		
cod		
Crab		
Herring		
Lobster		

Dairy

Dairy products can be both useful and harmful to your health. Full-fat dairy products can cause acne and increase inflammation. It has been scientifically proven that consumption of dairy products should be reduced to a minimum after the age of 33.

What to eat	Eat occasionally	What to avoid
Non-fat milk	Rice milk	Whole cream
Low-fat milk	Skim milk	Sour cream
Coconut milk	Tofu cheese	Cream
Greek-style Yogurt	Parmesan	Hard cheese
		Milk butter
Fat-free plain traditional yogurt		Margarine
Cashew butter		Cottage cheese
Sunflower seeds butter		

Eggs

Eggs contain essential nutrients, proteins, lutein, and zeaxanthin, which reduce inflammation. Nevertheless, frequent consumption of eggs can cause allergic reactions.

Nuts and Seeds

Nuts and seeds are useful for heart health and are rich in fiber and nutrition. Do not eat them, however, if you have nut allergies.

What to eat	Eat occasionally	What to avoid
Almonds	Hazelnuts	Chocolate-covered nuts
Chia seeds	Cashews	Nut butter (sweetened/ unsweetened)
Flaxseeds	Peanut butter	
Pumpkin seeds		Macadamia nuts
Pistachios		Peanuts
		Pecans

Vegetables

The main source of vitamins on the anti-inflammatory diet is vegetables. However, not all vegetables are beneficial. Avoid starchy vegetables and ones that can cause allergic reactions.

What to eat	Eat occasionally	What to avoid
Sweet potatoes	Tomatoes	Potatoes
Yams	Tomatillos	Potato chips
Beets	Corn	Champignon
Radishes		
Watermelons		
Green beans		
Organic baked corn chips		

Sweet pepper		
Shiitake mushrooms		
Bell peppers		

Fruits and Berries

Fruits are rich in vitamins. Nevertheless, avoid eating large amounts of sugary fruits. Replace them with sweet and sour or sour fruits/berries.

What to eat	Eat occasionally	What to avoid
Tart cherries	Kiwi	Acerola
Strawberries	Papaya	Lychee
Blueberries	Bananas	Persimmon
Apples		
Pears		
Apricots		
Avocado		
Dried fruits		

Orange	
Mango	
Pineapple	

Grain Products

Whole grains are rich in fiber and can combat inflammation and protect our body from infections. Avoid eating "bad" grains.

What to eat	What to avoid
Brown rice	White rice
Wild rice	Sugary cereals
Oatmeal	White bread
Whole-grain bread	Crackers
Multigrain bread	Snacks
Whole-grain pasta	Rye bread

Oat flour	Wheat noodles
Buckwheat flour	White bread crumbs
Whole wheat flour	Cornflour
Rice noodles	Wheat tortillas
Corn tortillas	Bagels
Whole-grain toast	

Condiments

Condiments play a significant role in the taste of a meal. They can make it tender, spicy, or salty. On the anti-inflammatory diet, you can use almost all spices and herbs. They have strong anti-inflammatory properties.

What to eat	What to avoid
Low-fat mayonnaise	Mayonnaise (full-fat)
Ground pink peppercorns	Tartar sauce
Turmeric tahini dressing	Teriyaki
Alfredo sauce	Tomato sauce
Hot red pepper sauce	Bordelaise sauce
Turmeric tahini dressing	Brown sauce
Chimichurri sauce	Chili sauce
Curry powder	Dijon sauce
Tapatio sauce (handmade)	Buffalo sauce
Apple cider vinegar	Hollandaise sauce

Pomegranate sauce	Marinara sauce
	Worcestershire sauce
	Sweet and sour sauce
	Soy sauce
	Pickle relish
	Barbecue sauce
	Dijon mustard

Oils and fats

It is recommended to consume vegetable oils and fats on the anti-inflammatory diet. Bear in mind that some natural oils can cause allergies.

What to eat	Eat occasionally	What to avoid
Sunflower oil (cold-pressed)	Walnut oil	Coconut oil
Grapeseed oil		Palm oil
Olive oil (extra virgin)		
Flax seed oil		

Beverages

Drinking water should be a rule for you on the anti-inflammatory diet. Avoid consuming sparkling drinks and beverages that contain artificial sugars.

What to eat	Eat occasionally	What to avoid
Fresh fruit juice	Fresh juice	Coffee
Seltzer		Sodas
Filtered water		Wine
Mineral water		Sparkling mineral water
Lemon water		Carbonated drinks
Herbal tea		
Green tea		Sweet sparkling beverages
Mate tea		

Sweets

Fruits are the best sweets on the anti-inflammatory diet. They are rich in vitamins and contain only natural sweeteners.

Nevertheless, you can find a lot of sugar-free meals which are not inferior in taste to the most famous desserts.

What to eat	Eat occasionally	What to avoid
Honey	Stevia	Artificial sweeteners
Raw cocoa powder	Xylitol	Buns
	Brown rice syrup	
Fruit (allowed for anti-inflammatory diet)	Black chocolate	Candy
		Cakes
		Chocolate
		Cookies
		Custard
		Ice cream

Pastries

Pies

Pudding

Sugar

Tarts

Corn syrup

Beans and Legumes

Consumption of beans and legumes is very important on the anti-inflammatory diet. They are rich in fiber and contain a high amount of proteins. Besides this, they provide a lot of antioxidants. It is necessary to eat at least two servings of beans or legumes per week.

Note that beans and legumes can cause inflammation only if they are cooked in the wrong way. It is recommended to soak beans before cooking.

Others

Fast food and processed food are forbidden on the anti-inflammatory diet. Such food damages our gut system and reduces the protective qualities of our body and, as a result, destroys the immune system.

What to avoid

Fried foods

Processed foods

Top 10 Anti-Inflammatory Diet Tips

1. Avoid white food.

Avoiding white food such as sugar, salt, etc. can help to maintain and control the normal level of blood sugar. Try to add more lean proteins and high fiber food in your daily diet. It can be lean types of meat, brown rice, and whole grains.

2. An apple a day keeps the doctors away.

Add vegetables, fruits, nuts, and spices in your daily meal plan. Garlic, ginger, cinnamon, and lemon will help to boost your immune system and reduce inflammation.

3. Exercise daily.

Regular exercise can help to prevent inflammation. Just 5-10 minutes of activity daily can help you feel healthier.

4. Balance your mind.

Everyday stress leads to chronic disease. Practicing yoga, meditation, or biofeedback are excellent ways to balance your mind and manage stress.

5. Choose the right proteins.

Lean red meat can be served as a source of proteins but is high in cholesterol and salt. Instead, choose fish such as halibut, salmon, tuna, cod, or seabass, which are rich in omega-3 fatty acids.

6. Drink antioxidant beverages.

Herbs are a great source of antioxidants and promote faster treatment. Basil, thyme, oregano, chili pepper, and curcumin have high anti-inflammatory features and serve as natural painkillers.

7. Control your sleep schedule.

Eight-nine hours of sleep should be a rule for you. Too little or too much sleep are the main triggers for heart disease and type 2 diabetes.

8. Eliminate alcohol from your diet.

Eliminating alcohol helps to keep the body calm and reduces the risk of inflammation.

9. Choose green tea instead of coffee or black tea.

Green tea can fight free radical damage. Regular drinking of green tea lowers the risk of cancer and Alzheimer's disease.

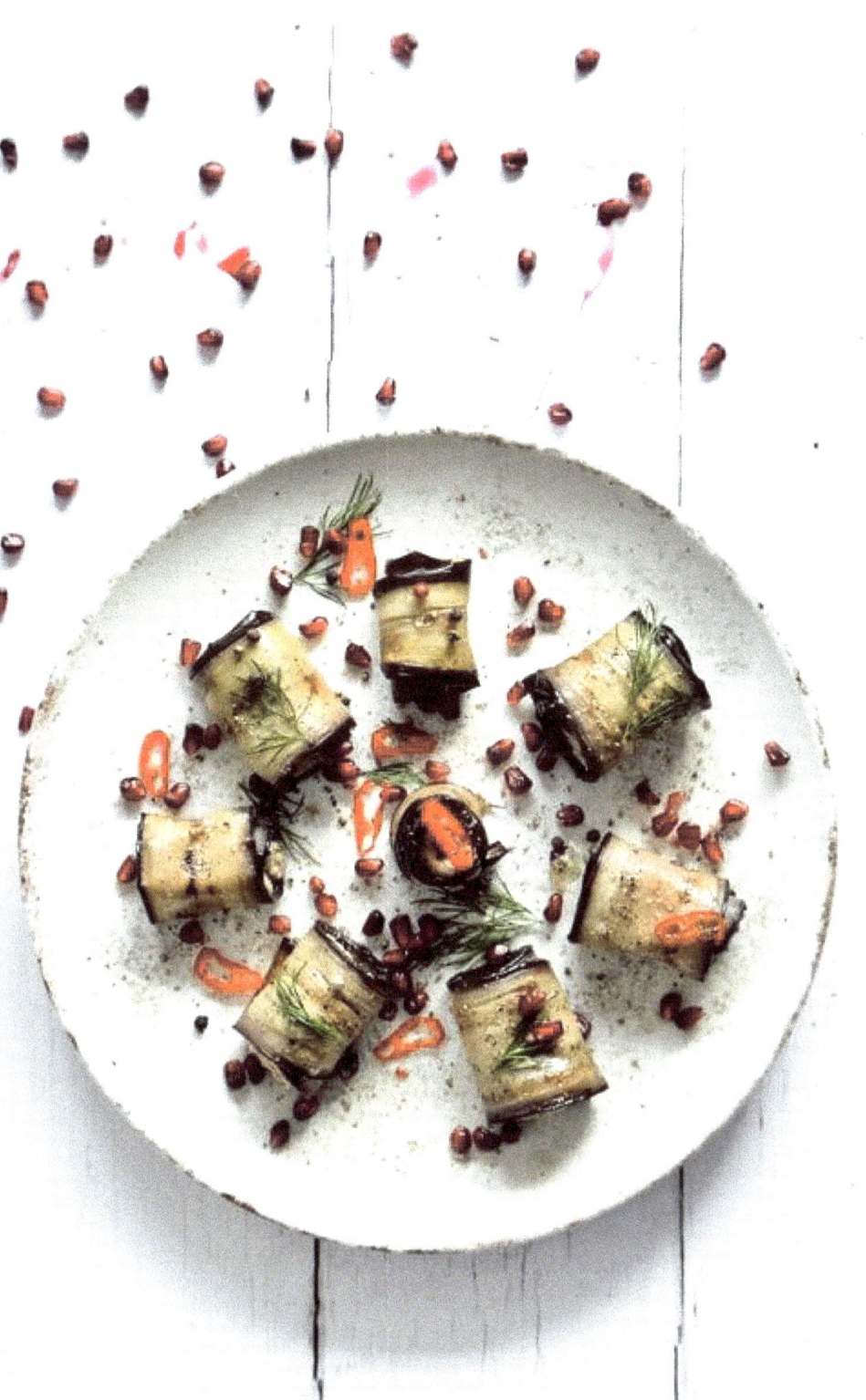

BREAKFAST

Spinach Frittata

4 Servings

Preparation time: 40 minutes

Ingredients:

- 2 cups spinach, chopped
- 6 eggs, beaten
- 1 tablespoon cashew butter
- 1 teaspoon chili powder
- ¼ cup coconut cream

Directions:

- Mix all ingredients except cashew butter in the mixing bowl.
- Then grease the baking pan with cashew butter and pour the egg mixture inside.
- Bake the frittata at 350F for 30 minutes.

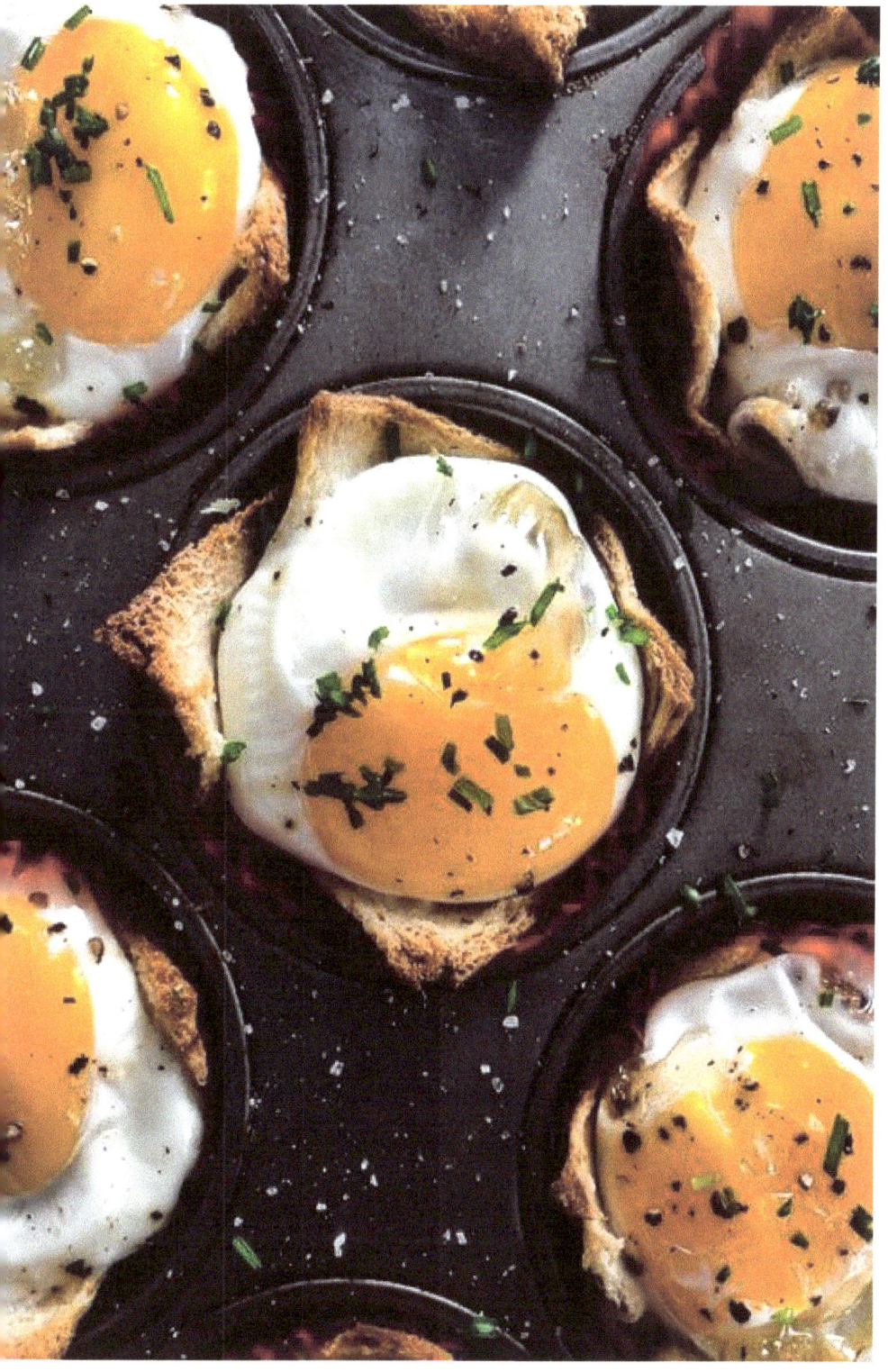

Granola Bars

4 Servings

Preparation time: 20 minutes

Ingredients:

- 7 oz pistachios, chopped
- 1 cup dates, pitted
- ½ cup raisins, chopped
- 2 tablespoons chia seeds

Directions:

- Mix all ingredients in the bowl.
- When the mixture is homogenous, transfer it in the baking paper and flatten it in the shape of a square.
- Cut the granola into bars.

Quinoa Salad

2 Servings

Preparation time: 10 minutes

Ingredients:

- 2 cups quinoa, cooked
- 1 cup tomatoes, chopped
- 1 cup fresh parsley, chopped
- 1 tablespoon olive oil
- 1 teaspoon lemon juice
- 2 garlic cloves, diced

Directions:

- In the salad bowl, mix quinoa with tomatoes, parsley, and garlic cloves.
- Then add olive oil and lemon juice.
- Stir the salad.

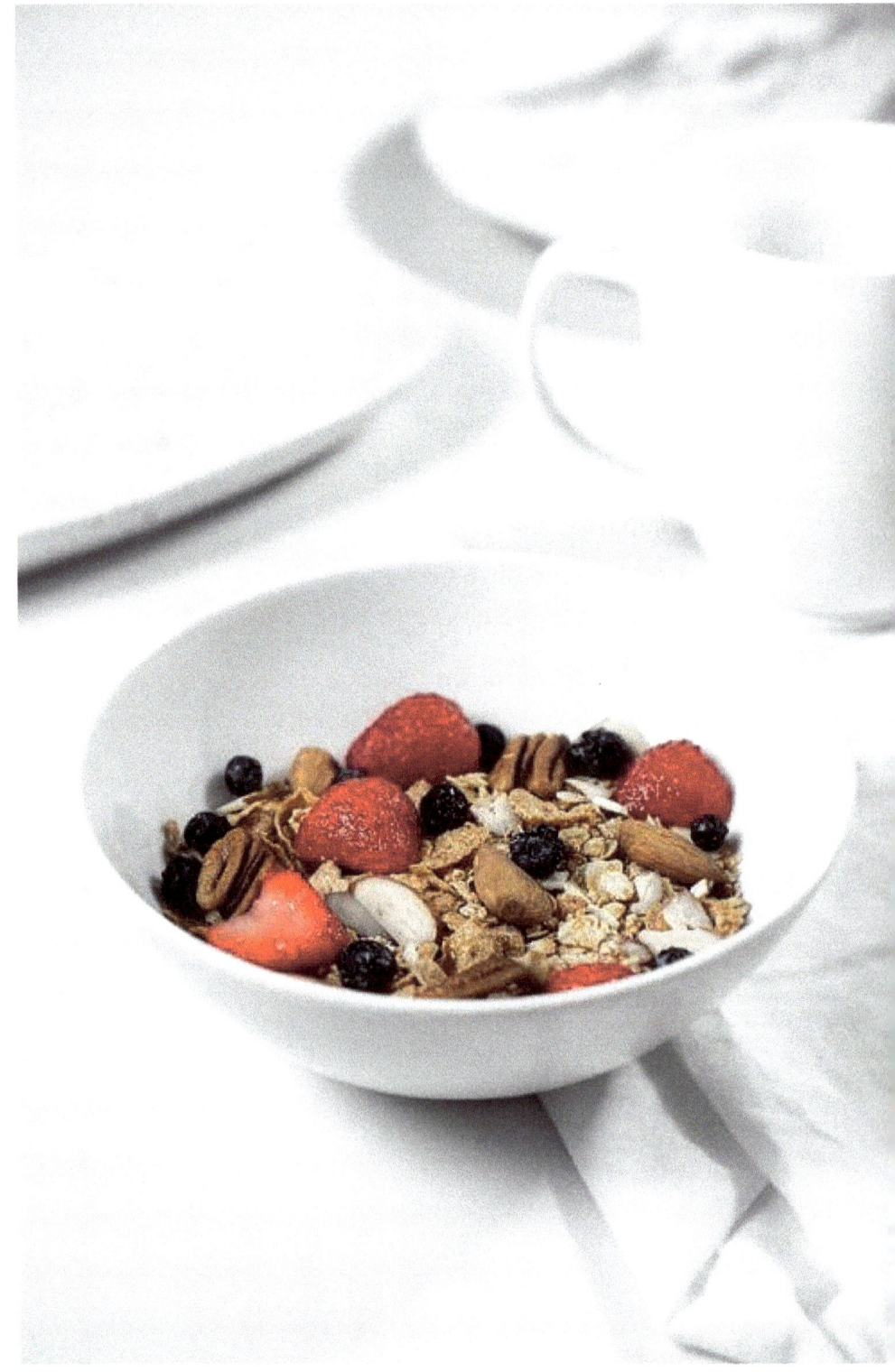

Shredded Carrot Bowl

4 Servings

Preparation time: 10 minutes

Ingredients:

- 3 cups carrot, shredded
- 3 oz raisins, chopped
- 3 tablespoons lemon juice
- 2 tablespoons olive oil
- 1 tablespoons dried cilantro
- 1 tablespoon raw honey

Directions:

- Put all ingredients in the salad bowl and carefully mix.
- Let the meal rest for at least 5 minutes before serving.

Italian Style Salad

4 Servings

Preparation time: 10 minutes

Ingredients:

- 1 tablespoon Italian seasonings
- 2 tablespoons olive oil
- 2 oz Parmesan, grated
- 2 oz olives, chopped
- 1 cup tomatoes, chopped
- 1 cup cucumbers, chopped

Directions:

- Mix olives with tomatoes and cucumbers.
- Then sprinkle the salad with Italian seasonings and olive oil.
- Shake the salad.
- Top it with parmesan.

Sprouts Salad

4 Servings

Preparation time: 10 minutes

Ingredients:

- 1 red onion, sliced
- 2 cups bean sprouts
- 1 cup fresh cilantro, chopped
- 1 tablespoon lemon juice
- 1 teaspoon dried rosemary
- 1 tablespoon olive oil

Directions:

- Put all ingredients in the salad bowl.
- Shake the salad well.

Corn Bowl

4 Servings

Preparation time: 10 minutes

Ingredients:

- 10 oz corn kernels, cooked
- 1 cup tomatoes, chopped
- 1 tablespoon fresh dill, chopped
- 1 tablespoon plain yogurt
- ½ cup radish, chopped

Directions:

- Mix tomatoes with fresh dill, plain yogurt, and radish.
- Then add corn kernels, gently stir the meal.

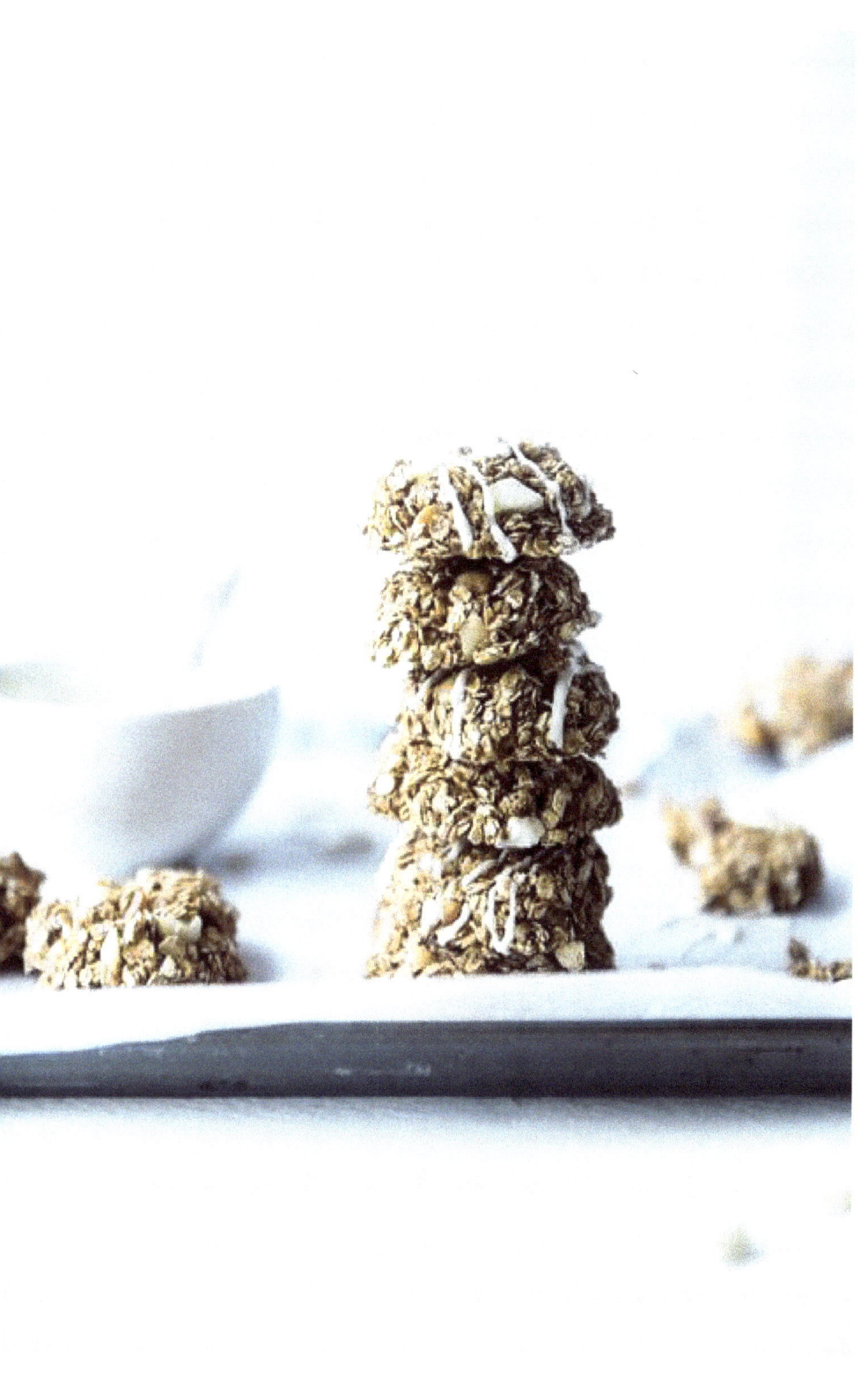

Lemon Tomatoes

6 Servings

Preparation time: 10 minutes

Ingredients:

- 4 cups arugula, chopped
- 4 cups tomatoes, chopped
- 2 tablespoons olive oil
- 3 tablespoons lemon juice
- 1 teaspoon lemon zest, grated

Directions:

- Put tomatoes and arugula in the salad bowl.
- Add lemon juice, olive oil, and lemon zest.
- Stir the meal gently before serving.

Avocado Salad

4 Servings

Preparation time: 10 minutes

Ingredients:

- 3 tomatoes, roughly chopped
- 2 avocados, pitted and chopped
- 1 cup parsley, chopped
- 1 teaspoon cayenne pepper
- ½ teaspoon dried rosemary
- 2 tablespoons olive oil

Directions:

- In the salad bowl, mix tomatoes with avocados, parsley, and dried rosemary.
- Then sprinkle the salad with olive oil and cayenne pepper. Gently shake the salad.

SAUCES, CONDIMENTS & DRESSINGS

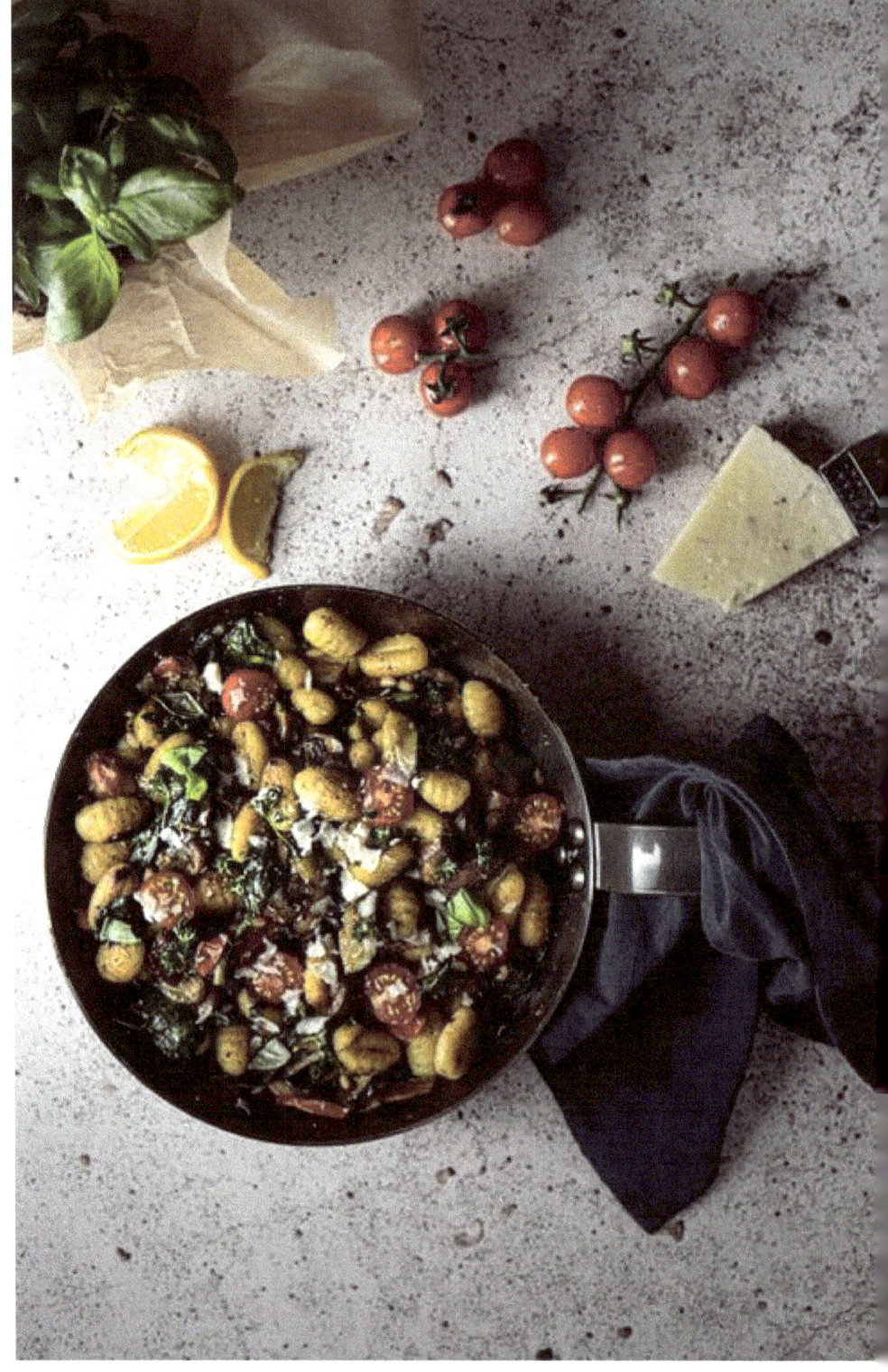

Garlic Dressing

4 Servings

Preparation time: 10 minutes

Ingredients:

- 1 teaspoon minced garlic
- 2 tablespoons balsamic vinegar
- 1 tablespoon olive oil

Directions:

- Mix minced garlic with balsamic vinegar and olive oil.
- Whisk the mixture.

Almond Sauce

4 Servings

Preparation time: 10 minutes

Ingredients:

- 1 avocado, pitted, peeled, chopped
- ¼ cup almonds
- ¼ cup of coconut milk

Directions:

- Put all ingredients in the blender.
- Blend the sauce until smooth.

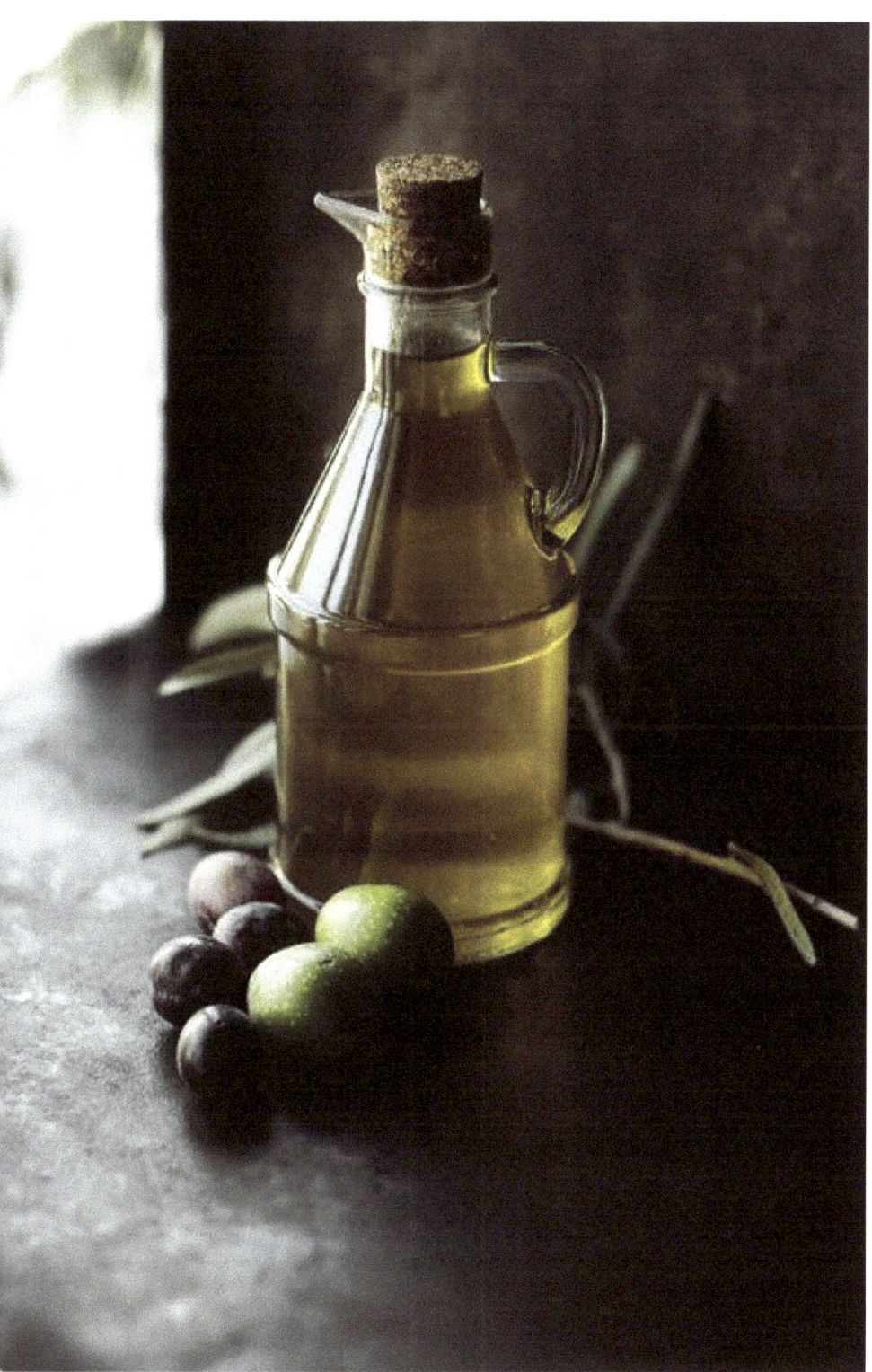

Sweet and Sauer Sauce

4 Servings

Preparation time: 30 minutes

Ingredients:

- ¼ cup lemon juice
- 1 tablespoon liquid honey
- 1 teaspoon chili flakes
- 1 tablespoon olive oil

Directions:

- Mix lemon juice with liquid honey.
- Add chili flakes and olive oil.
- Stir the sauce.

Lime Dressing

4 Servings

Preparation time: 10 minutes

Ingredients:

- ½ cup lime juice
- 1 cup fresh cilantro, chopped
- ¼ teaspoon ground nutmeg
- 1 tablespoon olive oil

Directions:

- Mix lime juice with fresh cilantro, ground nutmeg, and olive oil.
- Whisk the dressing.

Low-Fat Mayo

4 Servings

Preparation time: 10 minutes

Ingredients:

- 2 tablespoons mustard
- ½ cup olive oil
- 1 egg, beaten
- 1 tablespoon lemon juice

Directions:

- Put all ingredients in the blender,
- Blend the mixture until it is smooth.

Fast Salad Dressing

4 Servings

Preparation time: 10 minutes

Ingredients:

- ¼ cup of orange juice
- 1 tablespoon mustard
- 1 teaspoon raw honey
- 1 tablespoon apple cider vinegar
- 1 teaspoon dried basil

Directions:

- Whisk all ingredients in the bowl until you get a homogenous mixture.

Basil Vinaigrette

4 Servings

Preparation time: 30 minutes

Ingredients:

- ¼ cup lemon juice
- ¼ cup fresh basil, blended
- 1 tablespoon raw honey

Directions:

- Mix lemon juice with raw honey.
- When the liquid is smooth, add fresh basil and stir well.

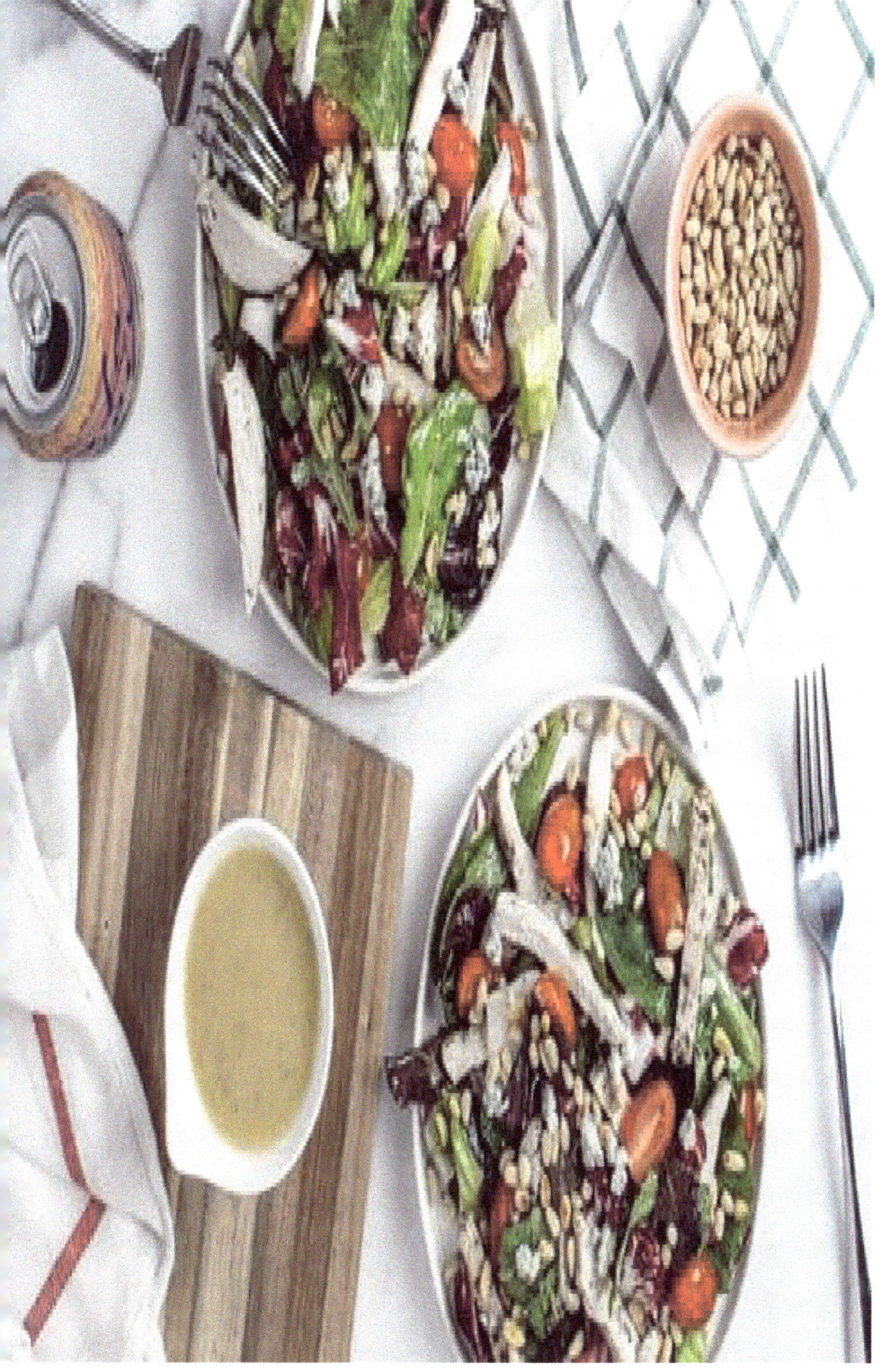

Lemon Pepper Dressing

4 Servings

Preparation time: 10 minutes

Ingredients:

- 1 teaspoon lemon pepper seasonings
- 3 tablespoons apple cider vinegar
- 1 tablespoon olive oil
- 2 tablespoons orange juice

Directions:

- Mix lemon pepper seasonings with apple cider vinegar.
- Add olive oil and orange juice.
- Whisk the dressing.

Creamy Dressing

4 Servings

Preparation time: 10 minutes

Ingredients:

- 1 avocado, pitted, peeled
- ¼ cup coconut cream
- ¼ cup lemon juice
- ½ teaspoon ground coriander

Directions:

- Blend the avocado until smooth.
- Then add coconut cream, lemon juice, and ground coriander.
- Stir the mixture well.

LUNCH

Honey Duck Fillet

4 Servings

Preparation time: 25 minutes

Ingredients:

- 1-pound duck fillet, chopped
- 1 tablespoon raw honey
- 1 teaspoon ground turmeric
- ½ teaspoon dried mint
- 1 tablespoon olive oil

Directions:

- Mix duck fillet with dried mint and ground turmeric.
- Then preheat the olive oil and put the duck pieces inside.
- Roast them for 10 minutes. Stir the meat from time to time.
- After this, add honey and carefully mix the meal.
- Close the lid and cook it for 5 minutes more.

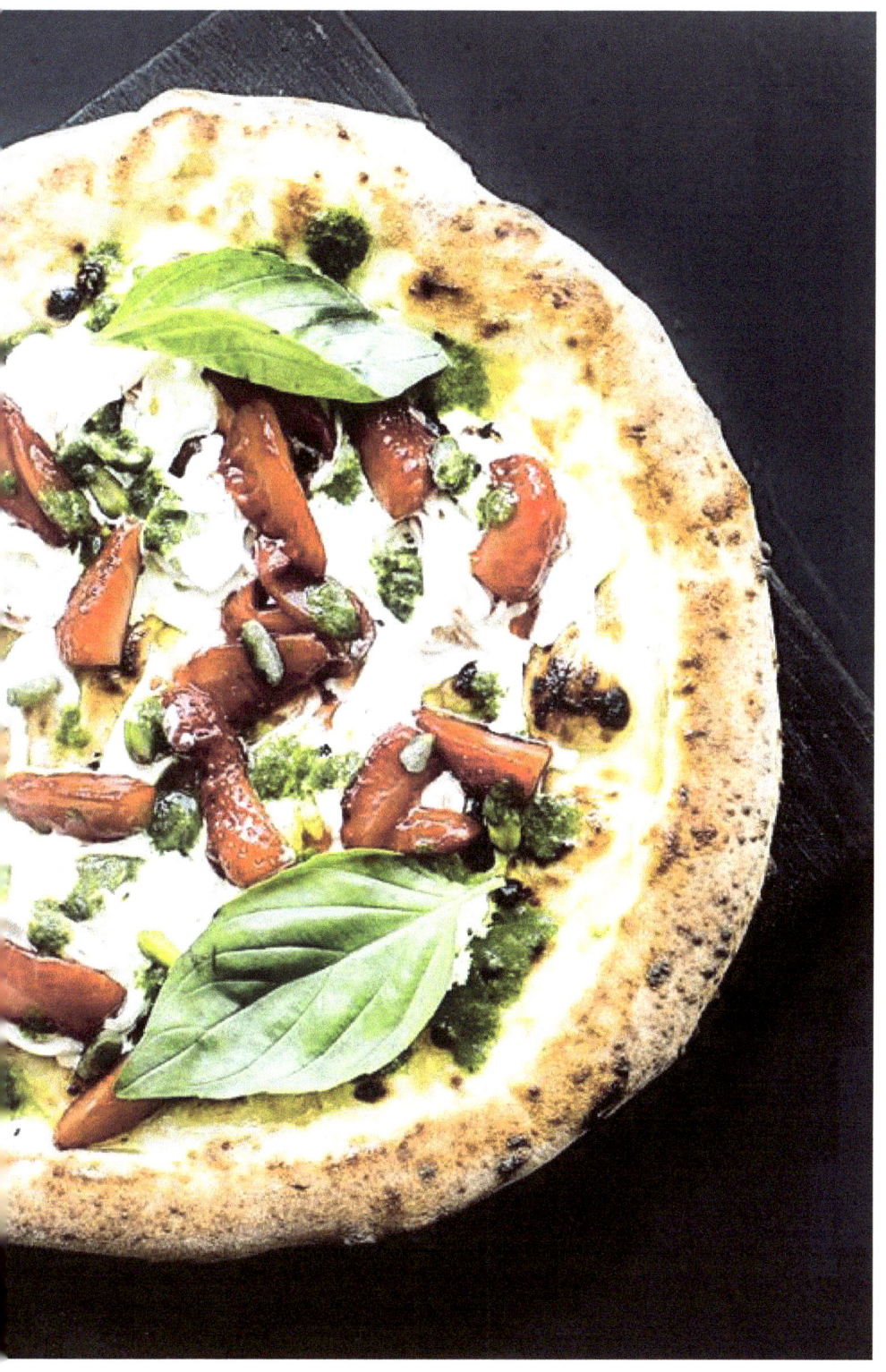

Sweet Chicken Bake

4 Servings

Preparation time: 40 minutes

Ingredients:

- 1-pound chicken fillet, chopped
- 1 cup peaches, chopped
- ½ cup of water
- 1 teaspoon ground nutmeg
- 1 teaspoon ground clove
- ½ lemon, chopped

Directions:

- Mix the chicken fillet with ground nutmeg and ground clove.
- Put the chicken in the baking pan.
- Add water, lemon, and peaches.
- Close the lid and cook the meal in the oven at 365F for 30 minutes.

Turmeric Chicken Wings

4 Servings

Preparation time: 45 minutes

Ingredients:

- 8 chicken wings
- 1 tablespoon ground turmeric
- 1 teaspoon minced garlic
- 2 tablespoons olive oil
- 1 tomato, crushed

Directions:

- Mix chicken wings with ground turmeric, minced garlic, and olive oil.
- Put the chicken wings in the baking tray, add tomato, and bake the meal at 365F for 35 minutes.

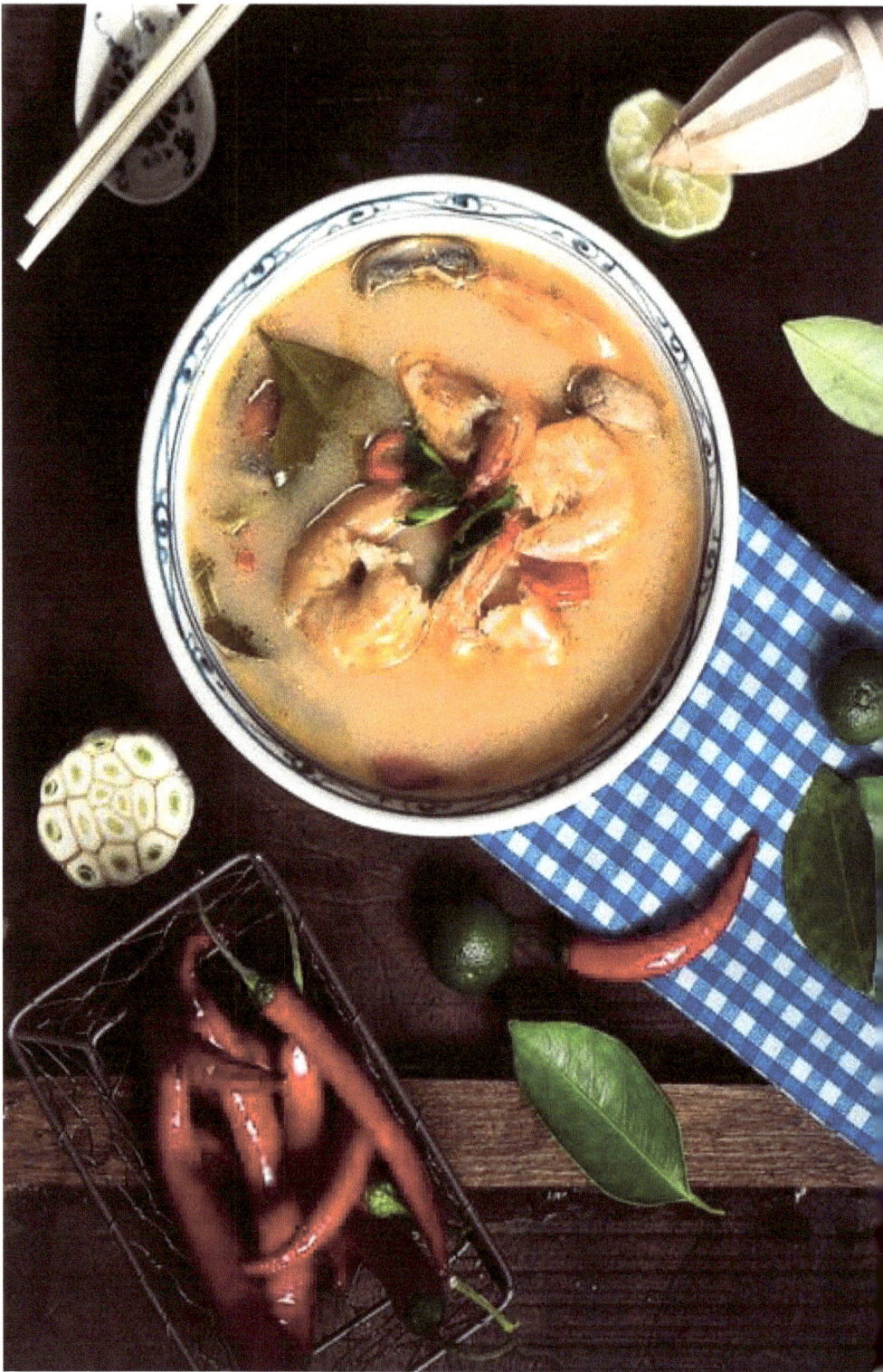

Salmon Meatballs

4 Servings

Preparation time: 20 minutes

Ingredients:

- 1-pound salmon fillet, minced
- 1 tablespoon minced garlic
- 2 tablespoons almond flour
- 1 teaspoon ground coriander
- 1 tablespoon olive oil

Directions:

- Mix salmon fillet with minced garlic, almond flour, and ground coriander.
- Make the meatballs.
- Preheat the skillet well, add olive oil.
- Put the salmon meatballs in the hot oil and roast them for 3 minutes per side.

Tender Chives Salmon

4 Servings

Preparation time: 15 minutes

Ingredients:

- 1-pound salmon fillet
- 2 oz chives, chopped
- 1 teaspoon ground turmeric
- 1 teaspoon chili powder
- 2 tablespoons olive oil

Directions:

- Rub the salmon fillet with ground turmeric, chili powder, and olive oil.
- Put the fish in the well-preheat skillet and roast it for 2 minutes per side.
- Then top the fish with chives and cook it for 1 minute more.

Parmesan Tilapia

4 Servings

Preparation time: 35 minutes

Ingredients:

- 1-pound tilapia fillet
- 3 oz Parmesan, grated
- 1 tablespoon olive oil
- 1 teaspoon chili powder

Directions:

- Line the baking tray with baking paper.
- Then rub the tilapia with olive oil and chili powder. Put it in the tray and top with Parmesan.
- Bake the tilapia ta 365F for 25 minutes.

Curry Trout

4 Servings

Preparation time: 25 minutes

Ingredients:

- 1 cup of coconut milk
- 1 tablespoon curry paste
- 1-pound trout fillet, chopped
- 1 teaspoon olive oil

Directions:

- Preheat the olive oil well and put the trout inside. Roast it for 2 minutes per side.
- Then mix coconut milk with curry paste.
- Pour the liquid over the fish and close the lid. Cook the trout on medium heat for 10 minutes more.

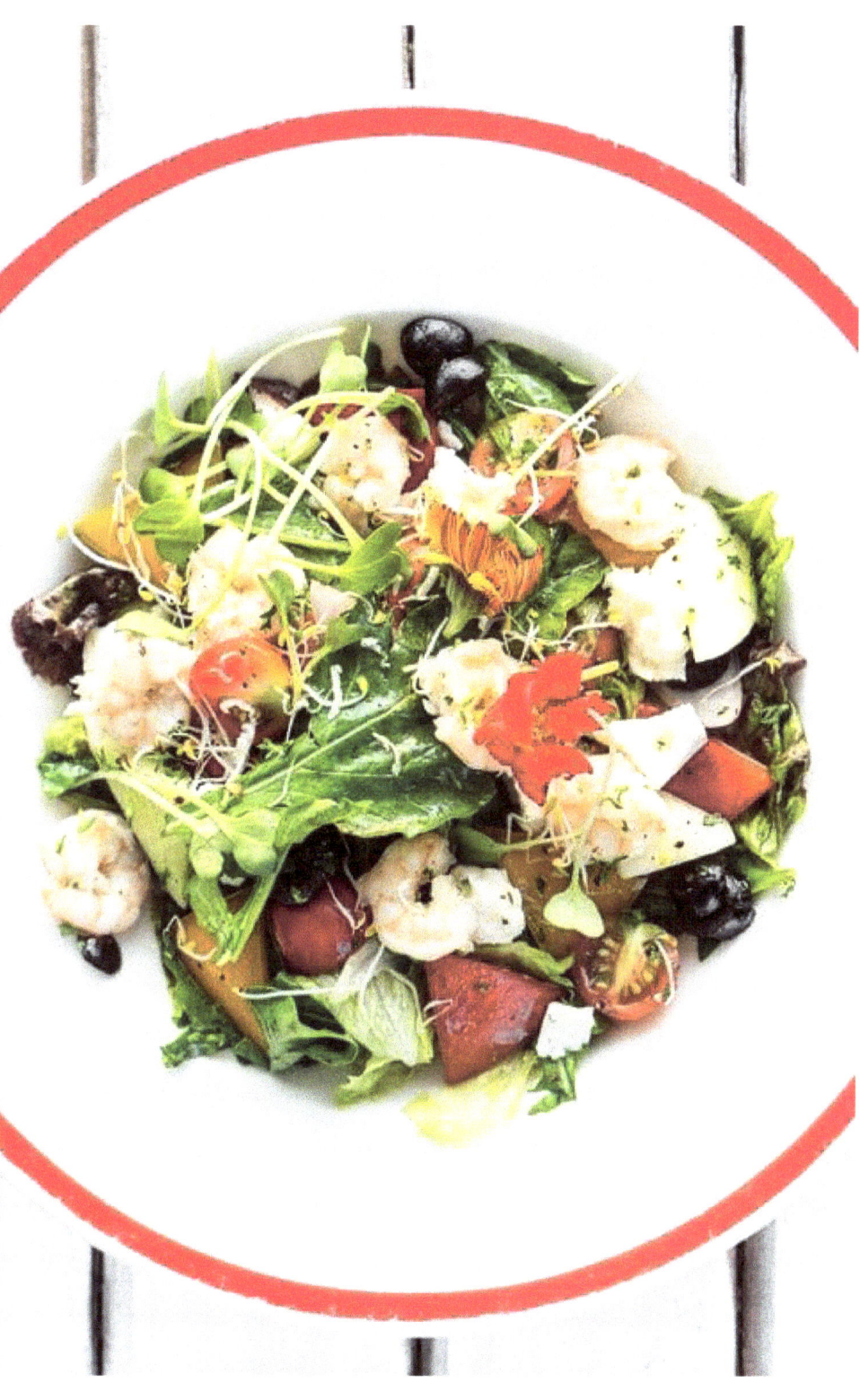

Lemon Crab

4 Servings

Preparation time: 16 minutes

Ingredients:

- 1-pound crab meat, chopped
- 1 lemon, chopped
- 1 tablespoon olive oil
- 1 teaspoon chili powder

Directions:

- Pour olive oil in the skillet. Preheat it well.
- Add crab meat and roast it for 1 minute per side.
- Then sprinkle the crab meat with chili powder and lemon juice and cook the meal on medium heat for 5 minutes more.

SOUPS

Coconut Soup

7 Servings

Preparation time: 35 minutes

Ingredients:

- 3 cups of coconut milk
- 4 cups of water
- 1 cup zucchini, chopped
- 1 cup broccoli, chopped
- 3 oz Romano cheese, grated
- 1 teaspoon chili powder
- 1 teaspoon dried mint

Directions:

- Pour water and coconut milk in the saucepan.
- Add mint and chili powder.
- Then add broccoli and cook the soup for 10 minutes.
- After this, add zucchini and grated cheese.
- Cook the soup for 10 minutes more.

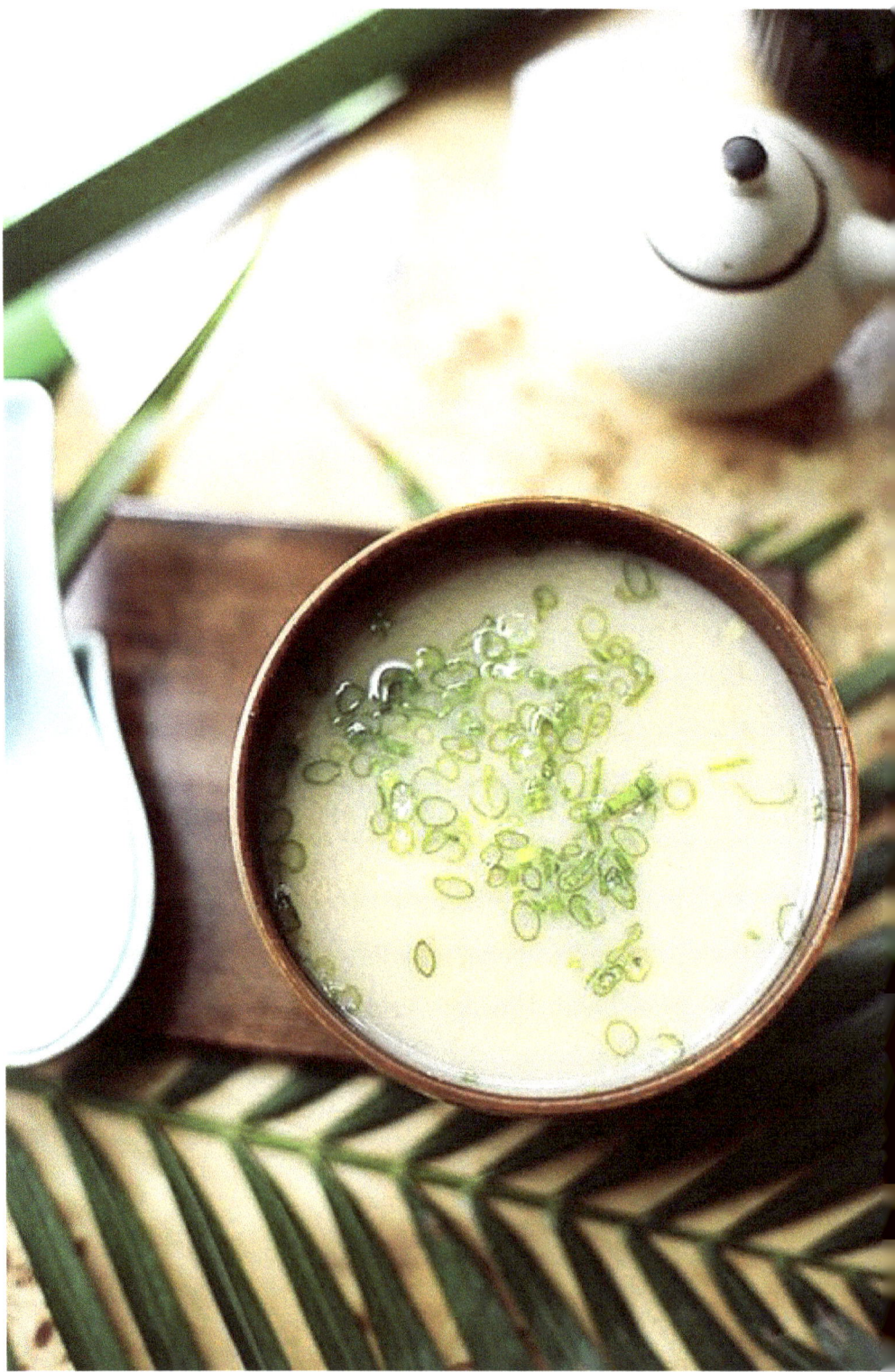

Seafood Soup

4 Servings

Preparation time: 30 minutes

Ingredients:

- 1-pound mussels
- 1 cup tomatoes, chopped
- 2 teaspoons minced garlic
- ½ cup fresh cilantro, chopped
- 5 cups of water
- 1 teaspoon chili pepper

Directions:

- Put tomatoes, minced garlic, and water in the saucepan.
- Add chili pepper and bring the mixture to a boil.
- Add mussels and fresh cilantro.
- Simmer the soup for 10 minutes.

Ground Soup

4 Servings

Preparation time: 35 minutes

Ingredients:

- 4 cups of water
- 1 cup ground chicken
- 1 cup leek, chopped
- 1 tablespoon olive oil
- 1 teaspoon ground coriander
- 1 teaspoon dried oregano

Directions:

- Mix olive oil with leek in the saucepan. Roast the mixture for 5 minutes.
- Add ground chicken, ground coriander, and dried oregano.
- Then add water and stir the soup.
- Cook it with the closed lid for 15 minutes on medium heat.

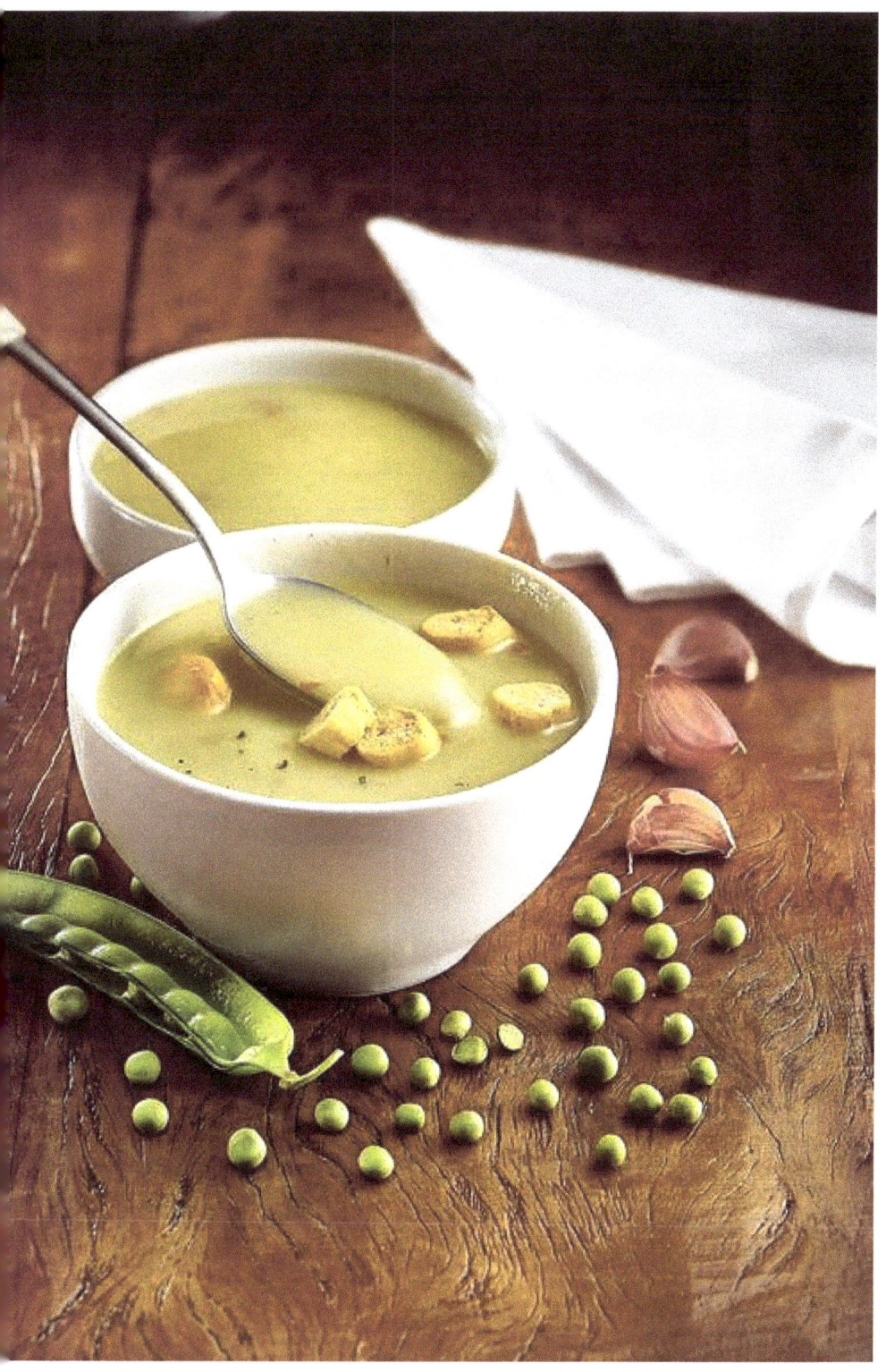

Rosemary Soup

6 Servings

Preparation time: 45 minutes

Ingredients:

- 6 cups of water
- 1-pound chicken breast, skinless, boneless, chopped
- 1 teaspoon dried rosemary
- 1 teaspoon dried dill
- 1 garlic clove, diced

Directions:

- Put all ingredients in the saucepan.
- Close the lid and bring the mixture to a boil.
- Cook the soup on medium heat for 30 minutes.

Cauliflower Cream Soup

4 Servings

Preparation time: 35 minutes

Ingredients:

- 2 cups cauliflower, chopped

- 4 cups of water

- 1 cup coconut cream

- ½ cup fresh dill, chopped

- 1 teaspoon ground clove

- 1 teaspoon onion powder

- 1 oz Parmesan, grated

Directions:

- Put all ingredients except Parmesan in the saucepan.

- Close the lid and simmer the soup for 20 minutes.

- Then blend it with the help of the immersion blender.

- When the mixture is smooth, bring it to boil one more time.

- Ladle the soup in the serving bowls and top with Parmesan.

Garlic Cream Soup

4 Servings

Preparation time: 40 minutes

Ingredients:

- 3 large zucchinis, chopped
- 1 cup coconut cream
- 4 cups of water
- 1 teaspoon minced garlic
- 1 cup pumpkin, chopped
- 1 teaspoon pumpkin pie spices

Directions:

- Pour water in the saucepan.
- Add pumpkin, zucchinis, and pumpkin pie spices.
- Add minced garlic and bring the liquid to a boil. Simmer the soup for 15 minutes.
- Blend the soup until smooth and add coconut cream.
- Bring the soup to boil and remove from the heat.

Bean Soup

6 Servings

Preparation time: 35 minutes

Ingredients:

- 1 cup tomatoes, chopped
- 1 cup white beans, cooked
- 6 cups of water
- 1 teaspoon ground black pepper
- 1 teaspoon ground paprika
- 1 onion, diced
- 1 tablespoon olive oil

Directions:

- Pour olive oil in the saucepan.
- Add onion and tomatoes. Roast the ingredients for 5 minutes.
- Add white beans, ground black pepper, and paprika.
- Stir the soup and cook it for 15 minutes on medium heat.

Sweet Potato Soup

4 Servings

Preparation time: 40 minutes

Ingredients:

- 1 teaspoon ground cinnamon
- ½ teaspoon ground ginger
- 1 teaspoon ground turmeric
- 1 teaspoon ground paprika
- 2 cups sweet potato, chopped
- 5 cups of water
- ¼ cup plain yogurt

Directions:

- In the shallow bowl, mix ground cinnamon, ground ginger, turmeric, and paprika.
- Then Pour water in the saucepan. Add sweet potato and cook it for 20 minutes.
- After this, add plain yogurt and spice mixture.
- Stir the soup and boil it for 10 minutes.

DINNER

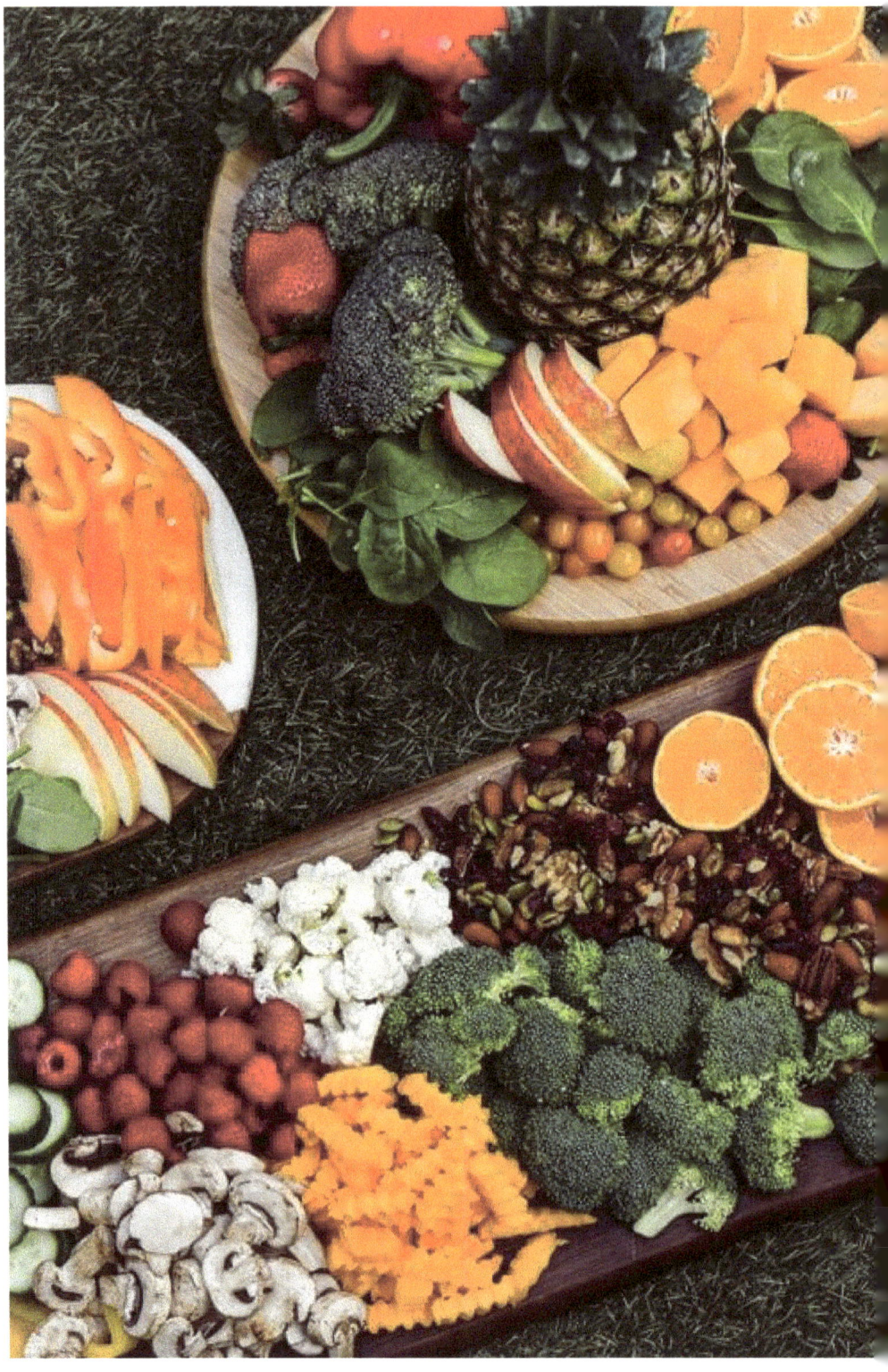

Cilantro Chicken

4 Servings

Preparation time: 30 minutes

Ingredients:

- 8 chicken thighs, boneless
- 1 tablespoon dried cilantro
- 1 teaspoon chili powder
- 1 tablespoon olive oil

Directions:

- Roast the chicken thighs in the olive oil for 5 minutes per side.
- Add dried cilantro and chili powder.
- Close the lid and cook the chicken for 10 minutes more.

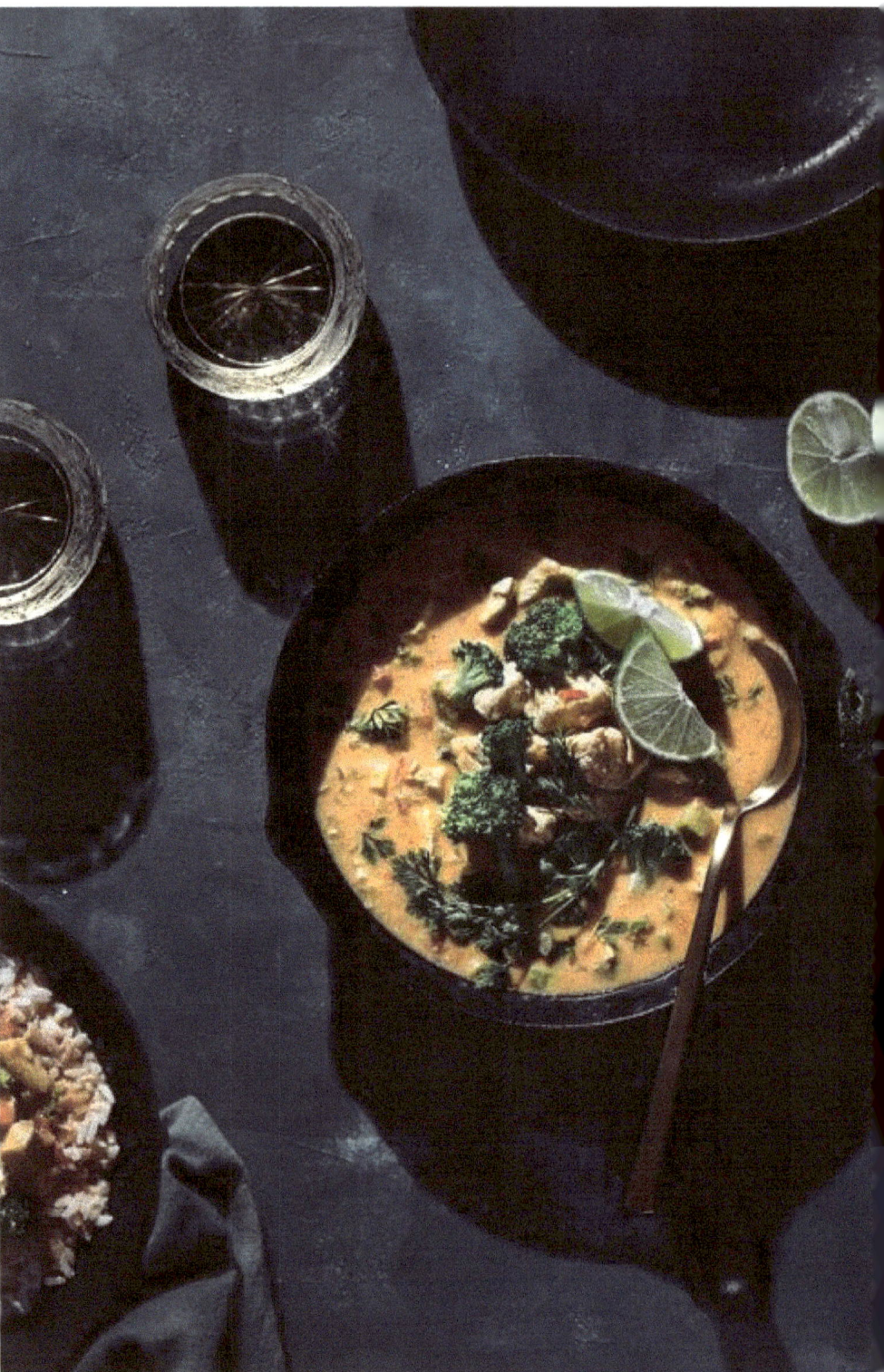

Jalapeno Chicken

4 Servings

Preparation time: 45 minutes

Ingredients:

- 3 jalapenos, chopped
- 1-pound chicken breast, skinless, boneless, chopped
- ½ cup of water
- 1 tablespoon minced garlic
- 1 tablespoon dried oregano
- 1 tablespoon olive oil

Directions:

- Mix chicken with minced garlic, dried oregano, and olive oil.
- Put in the saucepan and add jalapenos and water.
- Close the lid and cook the chicken on medium heat for 35 minutes.

Coconut Chicken Wings

4 Servings

Preparation time: 55 minutes

Ingredients:

- 8 chicken wings
- 1 cup coconut cream
- 1 tablespoon coconut shred
- 2 garlic cloves, peeled
- 1 teaspoon dried mint

Directions:

- Mix chicken wings with coconut shred, garlic cloves, and dried mint.
- Put the chicken wings in the saucepan.
- Add coconut cream and cook the meal on medium-low heat for 45 minutes.

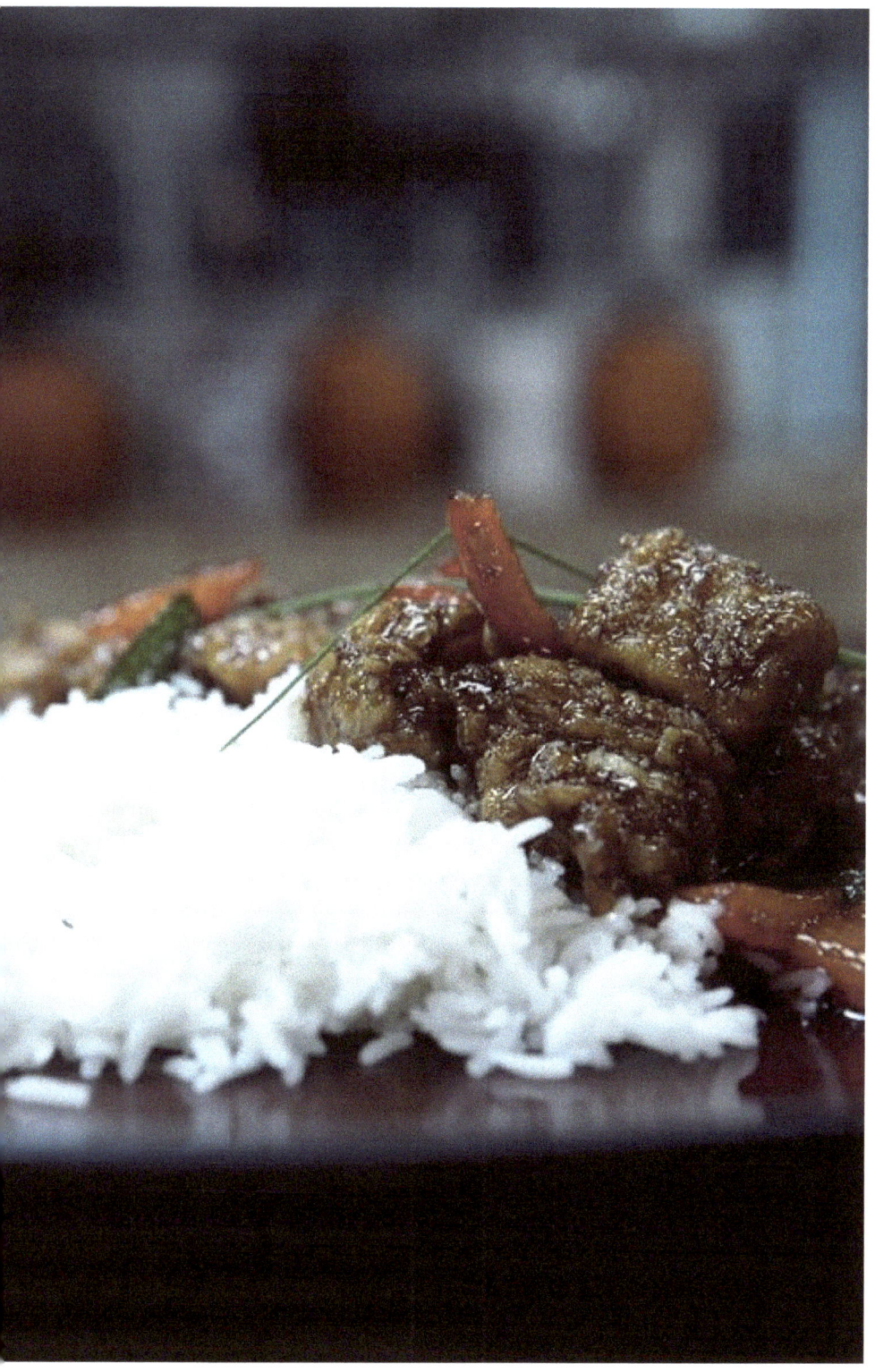

Corn and Chicken Stew

6 Servings

Preparation time: 45 minutes

Ingredients:

- 2-pounds chicken fillet, chopped
- 1 cup corn kernels
- 1 cup of water
- 1 teaspoon peppercorns
- 1 onion, sliced
- 1 teaspoon chili pepper

Directions:

- Put all ingredients in the saucepan and stir gently.
- Close the lid and cook the stew on medium heat for 35 minutes.

Chili Salmon

6 Servings

Preparation time: 22 minutes

Ingredients:

- 2-pounds salmon, fillet
- 2 chili peppers
- 1 tablespoon olive oil
- 1 sweet pepper, sliced

Directions:

- Preheat the olive oil in the skillet.
- Add sweet peppers and chili pepper.
- Roast the ingredients for 1 minute per side.
- Then add salmon and cook it for 5 minutes per side on medium heat.

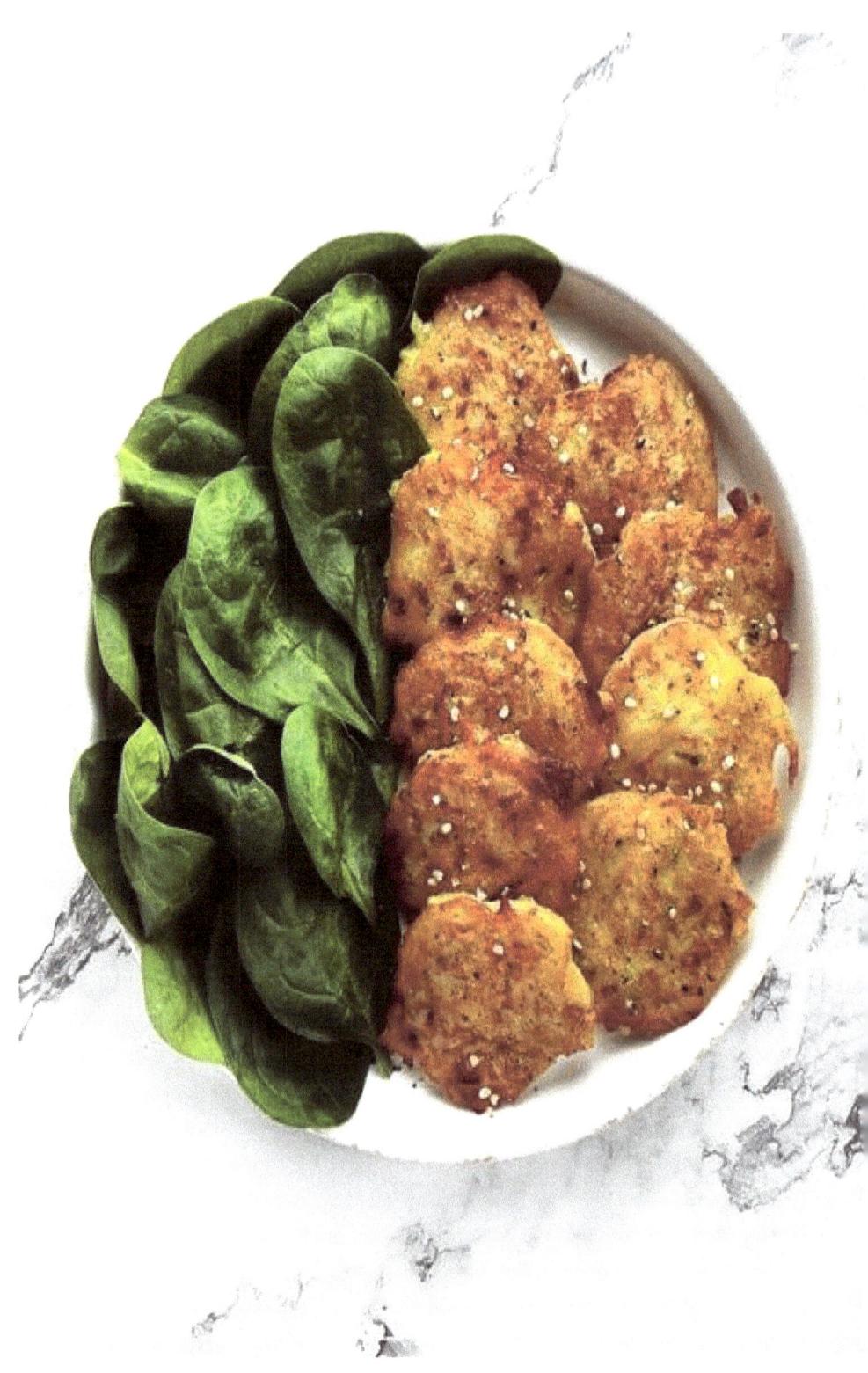

Garlic Clams

2 Servings

Preparation time: 20 minutes

Ingredients:

- 15 oz clams, cleaned
- 1 teaspoon minced garlic
- 1 tablespoon fresh parsley, chopped
- 1 cup of water
- 1 tablespoon olive oil

Directions:

- Bring the water to the boil and put the clams inside. Boil them for 3 minutes.
- Then preheat the olive oil well.
- Put the cooked clams in the hot oil. Add minced garlic and parsley.
- Stir the meal and cook it for 2-3 minutes.

Boiled Lobster Tails

4 Servings

Preparation time: 25 minutes

Ingredients:

- 4 lobster tails, peeled
- 1 cup of water
- 1 tablespoon dried rosemary

Directions:

- Bring the water to boil.
- Add dried rosemary and lobster tails. Cook the meal for 10 minutes on medium heat.

Turmeric Salmon

4 Servings

Preparation time: 20 minutes

Ingredients:

- 1-pound salmon fillet, chopped
- 1 teaspoon ground turmeric
- 1 teaspoon ground ginger
- 2 tablespoons olive oil

Directions:

- Mix salmon fillet with ground turmeric and ground ginger.
- Preheat the olive oil in the skillet. Add salmon.
- Roast the fish on medium heat for 4 minutes per side.

DESSERT

Sweet Grape Salad

4 Servings

Preparation time: 10 minutes

Ingredients:

- 2 cups green grapes
- 1 cup strawberries, chopped
- 1 tablespoon coconut shred
- 1 teaspoon ground cinnamon
- 2 tablespoons coconut cream

Directions:

- In the mixing bowl, mix green grapes, strawberries, coconut shred, and ground cinnamon.
- Top the salad with coconut cream.

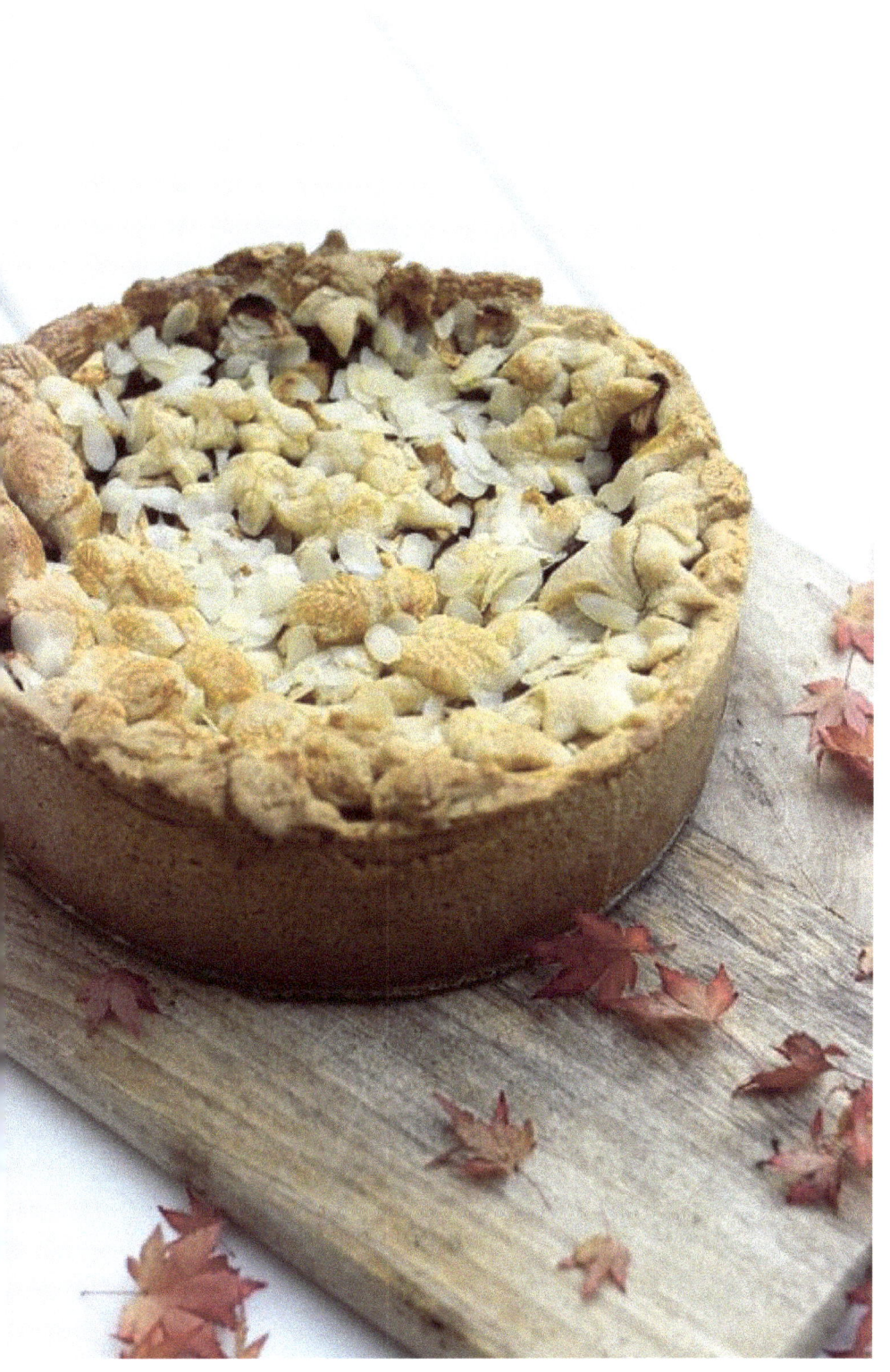

Mango Bowl

4 Servings

Preparation time: 10 minutes

Ingredients:

- 2 mangos, pitted, peeled, chopped
- 2 kiwis, peeled, chopped
- 1 cup watermelon, chopped

Directions:

- Put all ingredients in the bowl.
- Gently shake the ingredients.

Date Balls

4 Servings

Preparation time: 10 minutes

Ingredients:

- 1 cup dates, chopped
- 1 oz pistachios, grinded
- 1 tablespoon lemon juice

Directions:

- Blend the dates with pistachios and lemon juice.
- Make the balls from the date mixture.

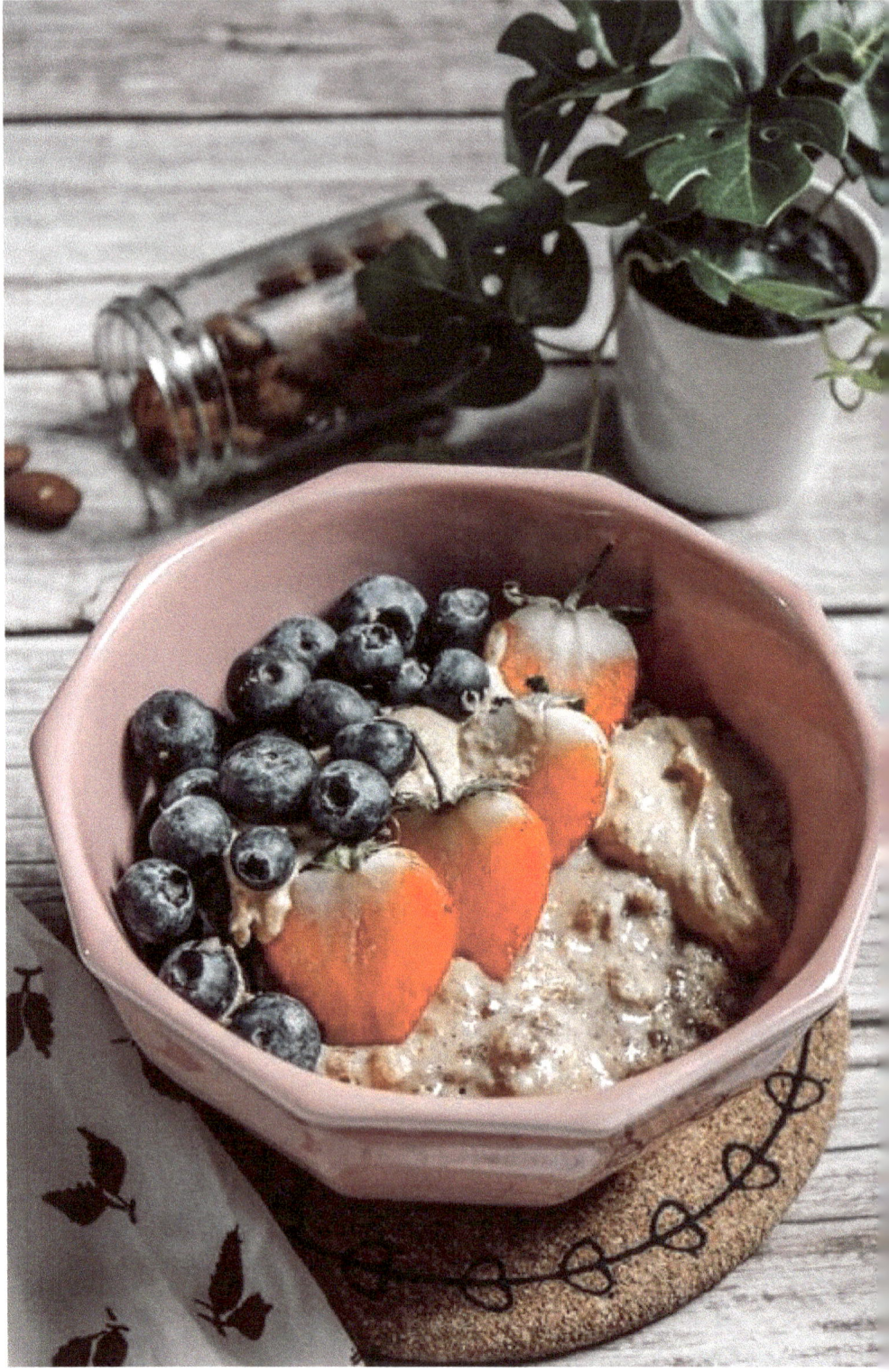

Baked Apples

2 Servings

Preparation time: 25 minutes

Ingredients:

- 2 red apples
- 2 teaspoons honey

Directions:

- Cut the apples into halves and remove the seeds.
- Then put the apple halves in the tray and bake at 400F for 15 minutes.
- Sprinkle the apples with honey.

Grilled Pineapple

6 Servings

Preparation time: 15 minutes

Ingredients:

- 3 cups pineapple, roughly chopped
- ½ teaspoon ground ginger
- 1 tablespoon coconut cream

Directions:

- Preheat the grill to 400F.
- Then sprinkle the pineapple with ground ginger and put in the grill.
- Cook it for 2 minutes per side.
- Top the cooked pineapple with coconut cream.

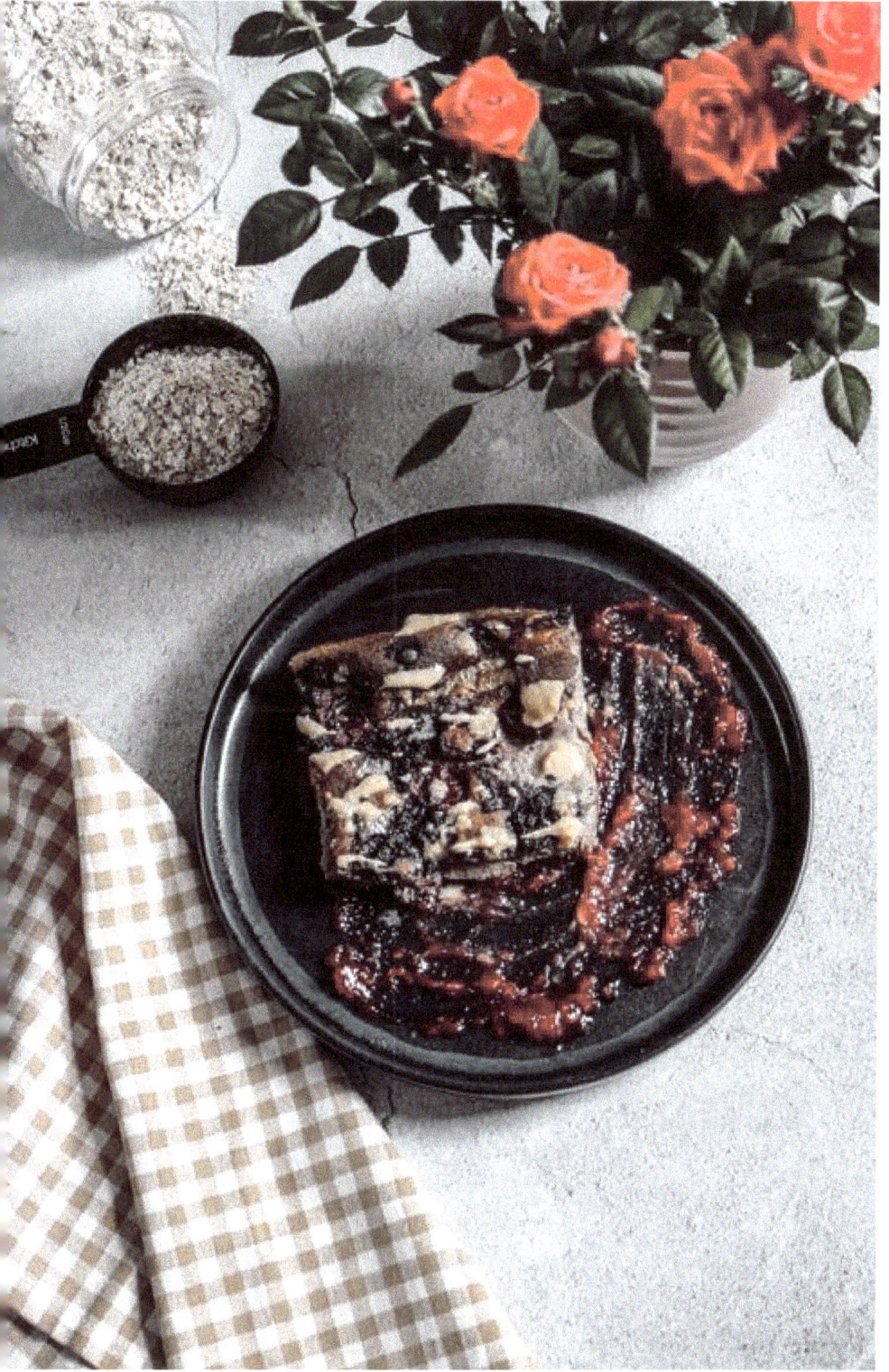

Coconut Shake

4 Servings

Preparation time: 10 minutes

Ingredients:

- 1 cup coconut cream
- 4 bananas, peeled, chopped
- 3 tablespoons coconut shred

Directions:

- Put all ingredients in the blender.
- Blend the mixture until smooth.
- Pour the dessert in the serving glasses.

Cinnamon Pears

4 Servings

Preparation time: 25 minutes

Ingredients:

- 4 pears, halved
- 1 teaspoon ground cinnamon
- 1 teaspoon raw honey

Directions:

- Preheat the oven to 400F.
- Then put the pears halves in the tray.
- Sprinkle the fruits with ground cinnamon.
- Bake the pears for 10 minutes.
- Then top the cooked pears with raw honey.

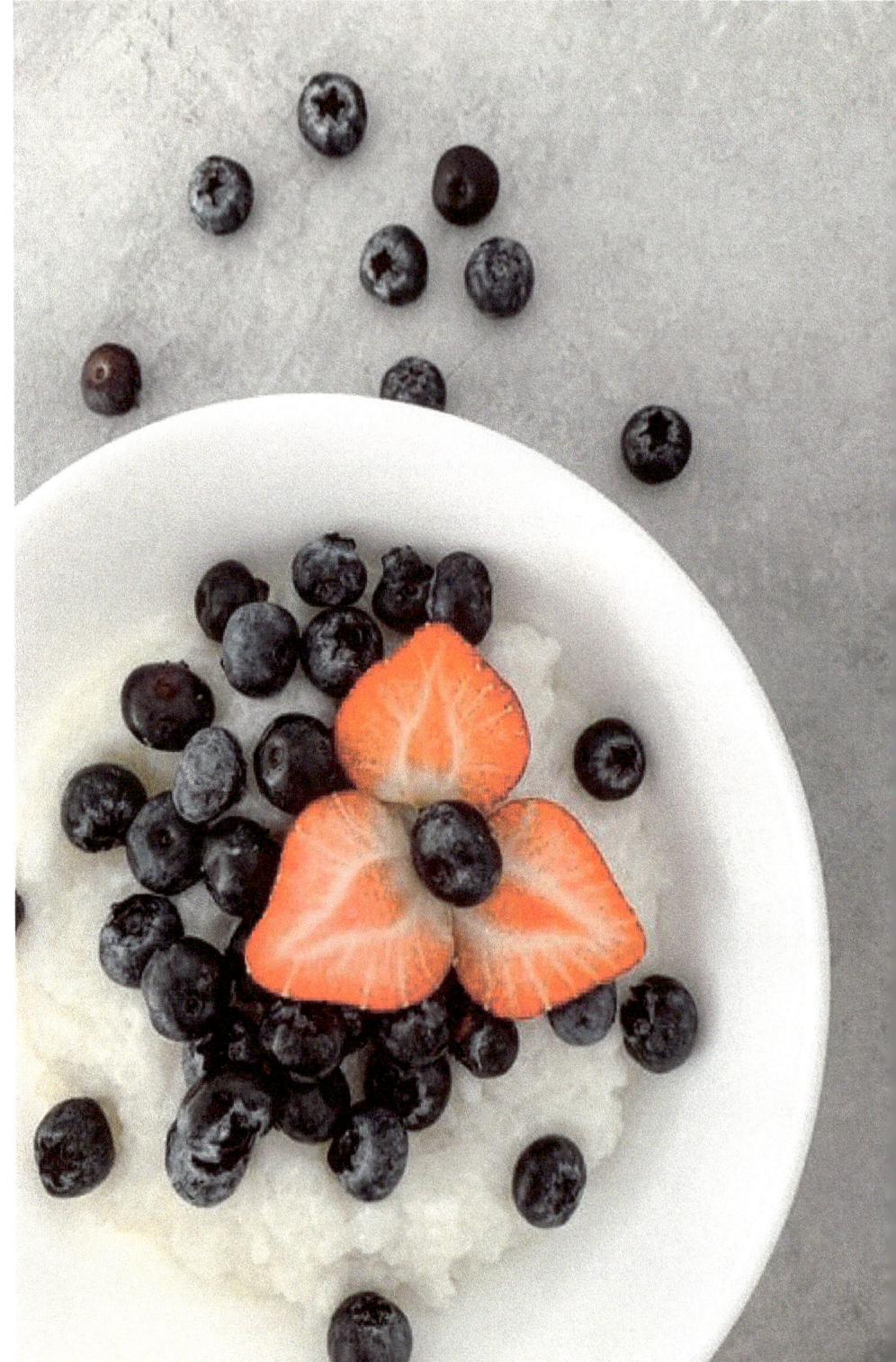

Melon Sorbet

4 Servings

Preparation time: 45 minutes

Ingredients:

- 4 cups melon, chopped
- ¼ cup coconut cream

Directions:

- Blend the melon until smooth.
- Mix the melon with coconut cream and pour the mixture in the plastic vessel.
- Freeze the sorbet for 40 minutes.
- Then blend the sorbet gently and put in the serving plates.

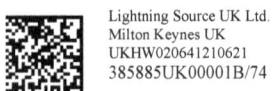
Lightning Source UK Ltd.
Milton Keynes UK
UKHW020641210621
385885UK00001B/74